Here is What Peop
Professor Medicare

As someone with a lot of office and insurance experience, I thought that signing up for Medicare would be something I could figure out for my husband and me. I spent a lot of time reading and re-reading the Medicare enrollment booklet. It's amazing how complicated and evolving it is. Luckily, I had saved a business card for Professor Medicare that I got a year before we became Medicare eligible. Donna Ludington of Professor Medicare helped us navigate the process, various providers and plans to come up with a Medicare plan that was the best fit for us health-wise and within our budget. Donna provides the kind of expertise and customer service that you hope for but never encounter. She answered every question promptly and thoroughly and when a mistake was made in our enrollment by Medicare folks, she acted as an advocate and got it straightened out the day I contacted her. We highly recommend Donna Ludington!

—Cheryl McLean- Boulder, CO

"As a program manager for an active adult community, Professor Medicare has been a regular and welcome presentation. The annual workshops have made a notoriously complicated government program not only understandable, but an enjoyable learning experience. The information conveyed has helped so many of my residents make the most out of their benefits and feel confident when making decisions about their plans. Resident feedback consistently praises the clear explanations and assistance with complicated situations. What an asset Professor Medicare has been for us!"

—Angela Harris, Lifestyle Director, Skyestone- Broomfield, CO

"Craig was GREAT!!!! He helped us to understand the whole process and pick out the plans that would be best for us. We could have spent weeks trying to figure out Medicare for ourselves, but Craig saved us all that time....and frustration and fear! I recommend him to anyone looking for info on Medicare! He is THE BEST!"

—Jane Jones-Arvada, CO

"He met me during dinner because I needed help quickly. I was new in town and needed a doctor. Craig has a great heart and is knowledgeable. He knows Medicare. Least of which this is not, I enjoyed my time with him."

—Michael Utz-Boulder, CO

I'm 70 years old and a seasoned professional in the computer industry, yet the whole Medicare maze really intimidates me. It has been such a find to work with Donna at Professor Medicare. Her many years of knowledge, and incredible attention to detail really compliment her kind and caring approach to each person she works with. I highly recommend Professor Medicare to get you through the maze and to the right side of the pathway!

—Nancy Allan- Broomfield, CO

"Craig (aka Professor Medicare) is the real deal: deeply knowledgeable about Medicare/insurance, extremely honest and highly competent. He was generous with his time, never rushing us and never aggressive about selling us a policy. He developed a keen understanding of our medical needs and identified the right insurance products to meet those needs. Better yet, he found a policy that saved us several hundred dollars per month over what we had been offered by my former employer. In short, he helped us successfully navigate into retirement by ensuring that we had the right health insurance. I strongly recommend Professor Medicare."

—Don Pemberton- Lakewood, CO

"Donna Ludington of Professor Medicare knows her stuff on Medicare. She was referred to me by a colleague I trusted. I contacted her for information On Medicare. She is a professional with smile, listened and answered my questions. If you need information before making any quick rash decision, call Professor Medicare and ask for Donna. There are so many reps out there pushing the products. Donna finds what is best for you. Doesn't that sound better than a salesperson? No obligation and free consult. So if you are thinking later this year to make changes in your healthcare, ask for Donna at Professor Medicare!"

—Nancy Chin-Wagner-Louisville, CO

Professor Medicare's Easy Guide to Medicare

MEDICARE IN PLAIN ENGLISH

Professor Medicare's Easy Guide to Medicare

MEDICARE IN PLAIN ENGLISH

BY

CRAIG STOUT AND DONNA LUDINGTON

Professor Medicare's Easy Guide to Medicare: Medicare in Plain English

Printed in the United States of America

First Printing, 2020

ISBN eBook: 978-1-7344161-1-4
ISBN Paperback: 978-1-7344161-0-7

Professor Medicare

1660 30th Street

Boulder, CO 80301

858-689-7445

www.ProfessorMedicare.com

prof@professormedicare.com

Ordering Information:

Quantity sales: Special discounts are available on quantity purchases by corporations, associations, and others. For details, contact the publisher at the address above.

Medicare has not endorsed, approved, or commented on this publication. We are independent insurance agents licensed to sell Medicare plans in Colorado and other states. Our intent is to clearly communicate a way of approaching and understanding Medicare. We have relied on the following government websites and publications to relay important information: Medicare.gov, CMS.gov, and 2019-Choosing a Medigap Policy: A Guide to Health Insurance for People with Medicare.

CONTENTS

INTRODUCTION

Most people dream of a relaxing, carefree retirement enjoying friends and family, travel and hobbies. But as it nears, big questions arise, creating anxiety about the future and waking us to reality:

> Do I have enough money to last 20–30 years?
>
> What will my quality of life be in retirement?
>
> What if my health changes?
>
> How much will healthcare cost?
>
> What will my relationships be like?

These questions can be distilled to *Money, Health, and Relationships*. We call these the *Big Three*. The Big Three concerns are inextricably linked and center around health.

As our bodies age, we may require more doctor visits, tests, medications, or hospitalizations—and their accompanying costs. Fortunately, seniors in the United States can rely on Medicare to safeguard both our physical and economic health.

Still, choosing a Medicare plan is like trying to order from a hundred-page restaurant menu. An alphabet soup of options ranges from Parts A through D to Medicare Advantage to Supplements. How can anyone decide what is best?

Well, when you don't know which entrée to choose at Chef M's (What is sriracha aioli? Will I like a deckle steak?), you ask your server for recommendations. When you need to make the best choice for your healthcare, ask *Professor Medicare.*

It's not just a cute name. At *Professor Medicare,* we have 10 years of experience helping thousands of seniors sort out Medicare's options. How? By translating the bureaucratic mumbo jumbo into everyday English and breaking the complex process into manageable steps.

Most of our clients are 65 or older and need healthcare coverage. Others already have Medicare but are unsure whether they selected suitable coverage. Some come to us confused and frustrated after attending lengthy "Understanding Medicare" seminars. But none of them wants to spend hours researching Medicare on the internet. They just want someone to point them to what they need and tell them how much it will cost. And that's exactly what we do.

We help you order confidently from the Medicare menu. As independent insurance brokers, we compare all the top Medicare Advantage, Medicare Supplement, and Part D plans in our area. Rather than shoehorn you into a plan, we find the one that matches your healthcare needs. And we make sure you understand what your coverage will protect, how much it will cost, and how to use it.

Over the years we have helped thousands of people dig through the mountain of information about Medicare and drill down to find the right coverage. Exploring and mapping that mountain has helped us streamline our process and make it easier to understand. Plus, listening to seniors from a variety of backgrounds and income and educational levels has taught us how best to determine each person's Medicare requirements. We discovered that individuals must address four primary questions, around which all other questions revolve:

1. When do I enroll in Medicare?
2. Do I stay with Original Medicare only and add a Part D drug plan? At what cost?
3. Do I enroll in a Medicare Advantage plan that includes/does not include Part D? At what cost?
4. Do I stay with Original Medicare and add a Medigap/Supplement plan and Part D plan? At what cost?

These questions serve as your **Map to Medicare.** Our job is to help you answer these questions and make that alphabet soup go down as easy as A-B-C.

This book is an expanded version of the process we use with our clients. We have gathered all our best professional advice, our clearest translations, and our proven step-by-step system into this single Medicare resource. Instead of searching online for answers or waiting for hours on the phone, you can find answers to all your questions in your own home at your own pace.

As you progress through the chapters, you will be guided to assess your own healthcare needs and knit together Medicare's patchwork of programs to make the best choice for yourself or your family. If you are an agent, this approach will give you a template for serving your clients at the highest level.

Let *Professor Medicare's Easy Guide to Medicare* serve as a trail guide on your journey toward understanding Medicare. Signposts along the way will keep you on track. Questions at the end of each chapter will be your mile markers, confirming your mastery of each topic. As our explanations clarify the options that are right for you, our gentle support will make the Medicare marathon feel more like a 5k.

A final note! We wrote this book and made it affordable so you can give it away. Please pass it along.

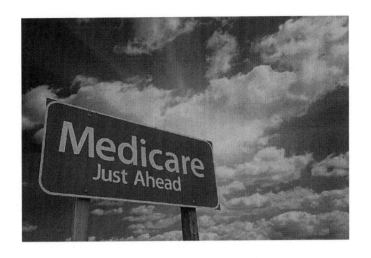

CHAPTER 1

A BRIEF HISTORY OF MEDICARE

Medicare is 56 years old. President Lyndon Johnson signed legislation creating Medicare in 1965, saying, "No longer will older Americans be denied the healing miracle of modern medicine."[1] Since then Medicare has given millions of seniors not only access to critical medical care but protection from financial devastation due to illness.

The program was expanded in 1972 to cover people with permanent disabilities. Medicare rivals Social Security in popularity, with 95% of more than 60 million beneficiaries giving their coverage a positive rating. But it took years of contentious debate for Medicare to become a reality.

---

[1] L. B. Johnson, "Remarks with President Truman at the Signing in Independence of the Medicare Bill," *Social Security: History,* July 30, 1965, https://www.ssa.gov/history/lbjstmts.html.

THE LONG, HARD STRUGGLE FOR HEALTH INSURANCE

Aggressive opposition from private medical insurance stakeholders led President Franklin Roosevelt to remove the provision for healthcare from his 1935 Social Security initiative lest it sink the entire package.

Years later Presidents Harry Truman and John Kennedy actively stumped for national health insurance, the latter saying, "We are behind every country, pretty nearly, in Europe, in this matter of medical care for our citizens."

Both received considerable pushback from the American Medical Association, which called it "socialized medicine," and from fiscal conservatives in their own party. House Ways and Means Committee Chairman Wilbur Mills thwarted Kennedy by holding up the bill in committee for six years.

Finally, the re-election of President Lyndon Johnson in 1964 swept in a liberal Democratic Congress. A compromise bill was developed that gave each faction a voice, and in 1965 America welcomed Medicare Parts A and B and Medicaid.

MEDICARE THEN AND NOW

The initial version of Medicare was much different from our current offerings. Then, if you were 65, a monthly $3 premium provided you only Part A, hospital insurance. Part B, physician and outpatient services, was optional.

Now, both Part A and Part B are mandatory.

PART A COVERS

- Inpatient hospital care

- Skilled nursing facility care
- In-home health care
- Hospice care
- And much more

PART B COVERS

- Doctor visits
- Physical therapy
- X-rays
- Diagnostic testing
- Outpatient surgery
- In-office injections/infusions
- And much more

Medigap, private supplemental insurance, is available to offset costs of Parts A and B. Beneficiaries may also enroll in optional private health plans through Part C, the Medicare Advantage Program, and Part D, which covers prescription costs.

FUNDING

Funding for Medicare Part A in 1965 came from a .35% payroll tax matched by employers. The next year that payroll tax grew to .5%, and in 1986 Congress raised it to 1.45% for employed workers and 2.9% for the self-employed.

Today, Part A is funded by a 1.45% payroll tax matched by employers. Parts B, C, and D are funded by a combination of general revenues, payroll taxes, beneficiary premiums, and state payments.[2]

Those payments go into one of two Medicare trust funds administered by the Centers for Medicare and Medicaid Services (CMS), which manages Medicare. CMS is a branch of the Department of Health and Human Services.

The Hospital Insurance Trust Fund is the repository for Part A payroll taxes paid by employers, employees, and the self-employed. Additional funds come from interest earned by the trust fund and Part A premiums paid by people who don't qualify for premium-free Part A.

The Supplementary Medical Insurance Trust Fund receives funds authorized by Congress and premiums from Part B medical insurance enrollees and Part D drug coverage enrollees. It also earns interest from trust fund investments.

PROTECTING MEDICARE

You might think Medicare's nearly-perfect approval rating and the peace of mind it has created for millions of seniors and people with disabilities would guarantee universal support for its continuation for decades to come. However, the program is expensive, and that makes it a target for presidential and congressional cost-cutters.

In 2017 Medicare's expenditures totaled $688 billion.[3] Growth projections put its outlay at $1,260 billion by 2028 due to

---

[2] "An Overview of Medicare," *Medicare,* Kaiser Family Foundation, February 13, 2019, https://www.kff.org/medicare/issue-brief/an-overview-of-medicare/.
[3] "Overview."

increasing numbers of eligible enrollees and rising healthcare costs.[4]

President Trump's 2020 budget proposed cutting Medicare by $845 billion over 10 years.[5] Members of Congress have suggested a variety of proposals for reining in costs, including privatizing Medicare, raising the eligibility age, increasing out-of-pocket costs, and expanding means-testing.[6] The Biden administration has talked about expanding Medicare as well as including dental, vision and hearing benefits in the scope of coverage.

All proposals to cut back on Medicare benefits should scare the bejeezus out of seniors, as the result will be decreased coverage and higher costs. Hundreds of people fought for decades to create Medicare. Now millions need to fight to keep it. We urge you to stay informed on this issue. Contact your members of Congress and let them know you want Medicare—and the seniors and disabled it serves—protected.

For more detailed information, go to *http://www.cms.gov* or *http://www.medicare.gov.*

---

[4] "Overview."

[5] T. Luhby, "How Trump Wants to Whack Medicare and Medicaid Spending," *CNN Politics,* March 13, 2019, https://www.cnn.com/2019/03/13/politics/medicare-medicaid-trump-budget/index.html.

[6] "Anticipated Congressional Proposals to Cut Medicare, Medicaid and Social Security," National Committee to Preserve Social Security & Medicare, January 16, 2018, https://www.ncpssm.org/documents/general-archives-2018/anticipated-congressional-proposals-cut-medicare-medicaid-social-security-2018/.

CHAPTER QUESTIONS

At the end of each chapter there will be five questions to help you retain important information that could impact your decisions for enrollment and coverage. Answers are in the Appendix.

1. When was Medicare signed into law?
2. Does Part A cover outpatient surgery?
3. What Part covers x-rays?
4. What organization oversees Medicare?
5. How can you help protect Medicare from cuts?

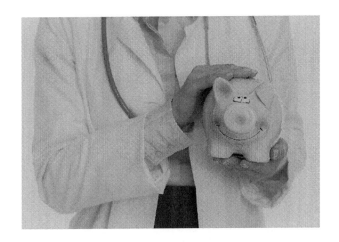

CHAPTER 2

PARTS AND PLANS AND TERMINOLOGY, OH MY!

"Parts and plans put pressure on patients to pick perfect provisions."

Whew! It's easy to trip over all those p's! Lots of people trip over Medicare's p's too, as it has both *parts* and *plans*. It can be difficult to remember which p word is which. Learning the difference is your first spoonful of Medicare's alphabet soup.

Parts refers to Medicare's areas of coverage. *Plans* pertains to extra insurance you can buy to supplement or replace basic Medicare.

So Medicare is divided into four *parts,* and you can purchase *plans* to enhance the benefits and reduce out-of-pocket costs for some of them.

PARTS

The least complicated aspect of Medicare is that it has 4 parts, simply labeled A, B, C, and D:

- Part A is hospital insurance
- Part B covers physician and outpatient services
- Part C includes Medicare Advantage (MA) and Cost plans
- Part D covers prescription drugs

Parts A and B are mandatory. Parts C and D are optional but may provide increased coverage and/or reduce costs. An analogy that may help you picture this is grocery shopping. Buying food for your family is mandatory. But you can choose the option to have your groceries delivered or shop at a discount store, which may save you time and/or money.

We'll go into more detail about Medicare's parts in the next five chapters.

PLANS

Plans are offered by insurers to bundle with or supplement Original Medicare. These include Medicare Advantage (MA) and Medicare Supplement (SUPP) plans. MA plans provide expanded services at low cost. SUPPs, also called Medigap insurance, pay for gaps in coverage when you use services or facilities. Basically, they reduce or eliminate copays and coinsurance. In Colorado, eight MA Carriers with multiple plans and nine different SUPP plans with around 40 Carriers will be offered in 2022.

This is an area of confusion—many people call us with questions about a SUPP, and we eventually learn that they mean MA or Part C coverage, not a Supplement.

TERMINOLOGY

Specific terminology is used in both parts and plans. You'll need to know these to choose and later, to use your healthcare coverage. A Glossary at the back of the book lists terms. These are the most common:

Premium: The amount you pay (usually monthly) for health insurance. Payroll deductions already paid for Medicare Part A, so you are not billed an additional premium for this. Your Part B premium is paid to Medicare. You may also pay premiums to other vendors for optional coverage such as MA, SUPP, or Part D drug plans.

Deductible: A fixed amount you pay out of pocket for services before either Medicare or your Medicare plan, or both, start paying.

Copay: A fixed amount you pay at the time of service. Example: You pay a $40 copay when you see a specialist.

Coinsurance: The percentage you pay when receiving a covered service. Example: An MRI may require 20% coinsurance. Medicare or your Medicare plan pays 80% and you pay 20% of the charge.

Maximum Out-of-Pocket (MAX OOP): The cap on the amount you must pay for services in a plan year. This doesn't include premiums but does include deductibles, copays, and coinsurance. After you meet the maximum out of pocket, your health plan pays 100% for the rest of the year.

SUMMARY

In this book, we will use certain terms over and over. Understanding the vocabulary, including knowing the difference between Medicare parts and plans, will go a long way toward helping you swallow that alphabet soup. Now that you know the terms, let's look more closely at Medicare's parts.

CHAPTER QUESTIONS

1. What is the difference between a *part* and a *plan?*
2. What does Part B cover?
3. How many Supplements will be offered in 2022?
4. What is a copay?
5. What happens after you meet your Maximum Out-of-Pocket?

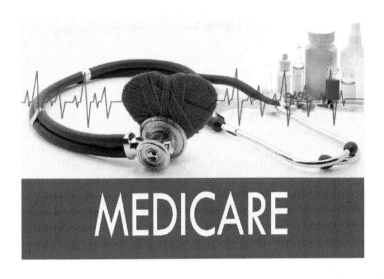

CHAPTER 3

PARTS A AND B:
ORIGINAL MEDICARE

"A little hope goes a long way," wrote Australian author Morris Gleitzman.[7] A little hope and a lot of hard work brought us Medicare. When it was first enacted in 1965, Medicare comprised only a mandatory Part A and an optional Part B. Since then, the program has indeed come a long way, expanding to include Medicare Advantage (MA) programs in Part C (1997), Supplements (SUPPs) (1980), and prescription drug coverage in Part D (2006). But Parts A and B, Original Medicare, still form the core of the program.

---

[7] Morris Gleitzman, *Then* (New York: Square Fish, 2013).

PART A HOSPITAL SERVICES

Part A covers you when you are admitted overnight to a hospital or skilled nursing facility. A simple way to remember it is that **A = A**cute care.

PART A COVERS

- Hospital stays and inpatient care
- Semi-private room
- Meals
- Skilled nursing services
- Special unit care
- Drugs, medical equipment, and supplies used during the stay
- X-rays and lab tests
- Operating room and recovery room services
- Some blood transfusions in a skilled nursing facility or hospital
- Inpatient or outpatient rehab after a qualified inpatient stay
- Part-time, skilled homebound care after a qualified inpatient stay
- Hospice care for the terminally ill, including medications for controlling and managing pain

PART A DOES NOT COVER

- Private-duty nursing
- Private room (unless medically necessary)

- Television and phone in your room (if there's a separate charge for these items)
- Personal care items like razors or slipper socks
- Long-term care
- Most care outside the United States

PART A COSTS

You have probably already paid for your Part A premium by making contributions from earned income through payroll deductions. Once you have paid Medicare contributions for 10 years or 40 quarters, you will owe no Part A premium. Individuals who don't meet that requirement are charged a Part A premium ranging from $274 to $499 a month. Exceptions are made for spouses who didn't work but whose partners did contribute.

Once you pay your premium, everything is covered, right? Sorry. Part A has multiple benefit periods per year, with (as of 2022) a $1556 deductible charged in each period. Many of you are used to healthcare plans with yearly deductibles. This is much different. Coinsurance adds more fees. These may accrue daily. In addition, there is no maximum out of pocket—no cap on your Part A out-of-pocket expenses.

Here is the breakdown for Part A in-hospital deductibles and coinsurance:

1. $1556 deductible per 60-day benefit period. This covers you for days 1–60 with no additional coinsurance charges.

2. After 60 days in the hospital, you pay $389 coinsurance per day up to 90 days.
3. Starting on day 91, coinsurance is $788 per day.
4. After day 90 you have 60 "lifetime reserve days"— that's for your entire life. After you have used the 60 lifetime reserve days, you are responsible for all costs.

For Medicare to cover you at all, you must be admitted to the hospital as an inpatient via an official doctor's order, which means the doctor says it's medically necessary that you have hospital care. Also, the hospital must accept Medicare.

From day one of your admission to a hospital, the calendar starts numbering days of your 60-day benefit period. A $1556 deductible is charged for this first benefit period.

Let's say you were admitted on March 1 and discharged after 3 days. If you are readmitted 30 days later, you will not pay another deductible, as your initial $1556 deductible covers days 1–63. However, if you are admitted again on the 64th day after your initial admission, you will have to pay another $1556 because you are starting a new benefit period.

It could get expensive if you have only Original Medicare (Parts A and B) coverage. Optional SUPPs and MA plans provide up to 365 days with different deductibles and coinsurance charges. More on these later.

PART B PHYSICIAN AND OUTPATIENT SERVICES

Part B covers medical and doctor services outside of the hospital. A simple way to remember it is that **B = B**asic, everyday medical care.

PART B COVERS

- Doctor visits
- Ambulance services
- Lab services including blood work and urine tests
- Preventive services such as colonoscopies, flu shots, and mammograms
- MRIs, x-rays, CT scans, EKGs, and a range of diagnostics
- Cardiac rehabilitation
- Obesity counseling
- Smoking cessation
- Mental health care
- Durable medical equipment such as oxygen, wheelchairs, and walkers
- Outpatient surgery
- Physical therapy
- Speech-language pathology services
- Occupational therapy
- Annual wellness visit
- Chiropractic services
- Injections administered in a doctor's office
- And more

PART B DOES NOT COVER

- Most prescription drugs
- Eye exams, glasses, or contacts
- Dental cleanings, exams, or x-rays

- Hearing aids

PART B COSTS

You pay your Part B premium directly to Medicare every month. For 2022 the premium starts at $170.10. In addition, Part B has a deductible of $233. After paying the yearly deductible, you will have a 20% copayment for all services.

Unlike Part A, this deductible covers the entire year. Like Part A, there is no cap on yearly out-of-pocket expenses.

SUMMARY

When you sign up for Medicare, you are automatically enrolled in Parts A and B. Part A covers hospital care and Part B covers physician and outpatient services. These provide basic health care at a reasonable cost. But as you have seen, Parts A and B do not cover everything and entail deductibles, copays, and coinsurance—not to mention the sky's the limit on yearly out-of-pocket costs. How can you improve your coverage while decreasing these costs?

Medicare Parts C and D. Next chapter.

CHAPTER QUESTIONS

1. When was prescription drug coverage added to Medicare?
2. Once you have paid into Medicare for 10 years or 40 quarters, what is your Part A premium?
3. What is the Part B deductible?
4. What covers you if you are admitted to a hospital?
5. Does Part B cover hearing aids?

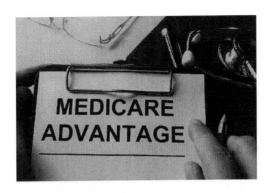

CHAPTER 4

PART C: MEDICARE ADVANTAGE (MA) PLANS

Original Medicare (Parts A and B) has been a boon for seniors and the disabled in reining in healthcare costs and providing a safety net against financial ruin due to catastrophic illness.

But subscribers clamored for options that would cover additional services and make out-of-pocket costs more predictable.

In 2003 The government responded with the Medicare Prescription Drug Improvement and Modernization Act, which created Medicare Part C. Part C plans would bundle Original Medicare with additional benefits.

Insurers created a Baskin-Robbins-like flavor array of Medicare Advantage plans offering services such as vision or fitness and reducing and/or eliminating deductibles, copays, and coinsurance. Most also included prescription drug coverage.

Finally, Medicare subscribers had real choices. This will help you remember what Part C does: Part **C = C**hoice.

Today approximately 34% of all Medicare users have MA plans. Each year, as benefits expand, that percentage sees an increase. About 60% of our clients choose MA plans. Let's look at how they work.

The Center for Medicare Services (CMS) approves and regulates all plans, which must follow CMS rules and regulations. Plans are approved yearly with a January 1 start date. Every September you will receive two reports notifying you of changes in costs, coverages, or your service area. The Annual Notice of Changes (ANOC) will detail any changes in your plan beginning January 1. The Evidence of Coverage (EOC) will list the details of your plan.

If you want to see if there are better options to your current plan, you can look at other offerings. Agents can discuss new plans after October 1, but enrollment must wait until the Annual Enrollment Period (AEP) begins on October 15. We see changes every year with every plan. Some are minor while others may impact your choice to stay with that plan. Also, new plans may come into your area and some may have attractive costs and benefits.

For example, in Colorado, we are added three new MA carriers for 2020.

ORIGINAL MEDICARE AND MEDICARE ADVANTAGE (MA)

Recall that when you sign up for Medicare A and B, you are enrolling in Original Medicare. Original Medicare has a schedule of "fee-for-service" charges that providers follow. If you visit your primary care physician, Medicare Part B will pay a fixed amount for that service. Same goes for any service from a hospital or provider.

With MA plans, which are owned by private health insurance companies, you no longer use Original Medicare. You won't need your red, white, and blue Medicare card, so file it safely away. You will be issued a card from an insurance company and it will be the one you use at providers and for your prescriptions.

Each MA insurance carrier has a contract with CMS and is paid around $900 monthly for your membership, regardless of your volume of usage or health condition. It is up to the carrier to contract with providers, hospitals, and pharmacies.

There are a variety of MA plans. In Colorado, most of our enrollments are in Health Maintenance Organizations (HMOs) and Preferred Provider Organizations (PPOs). But there are others, and we will list each with a short explanation. Keep in mind that around 95% of all MA subscribers use HMOs and PPOs.

STAR RATINGS

CMS assigns star ratings to each MA based on more than 50 criteria including preventive medicine, customer service, appeals and grievances, and quality of care. Plans are given financial bonuses for achieving over three stars. If a plan rates fewer than three stars for three years in a row, it is called "low-performing." You can join a five-star plan at any time during the year.

Clients often ask us which plans are the best overall. Star ratings are important in that they separate good performers from lesser plans. However, we have found that clients pay much more attention to costs and benefits if an MA's star rating is comparable to other plans in the area.

MA HEALTH MAINTENANCE ORGANIZATIONS (HMO)

Each HMO plan has a specific network whose providers you must use in order to get the published rates for services. You may however, obtain out-of-area emergency care, urgent care, or dialysis from non-network providers. Under their managed-care model, HMOs require you to choose a primary care physician, and you need a referral to see a specialist or for tests or lab work. There are a few exceptions. One of our carriers is an HMO but doesn't require a referral to see an in-network specialist.

If you live in a metropolitan area with an established HMO, the network will usually be robust with an extensive list of doctors and facilities. If you are in a less populated area, the choices are slimmer.

Many HMOs have no monthly premium. That means your only premium cost would be $170.10 (income based) for Part B. Plus, most HMOs have no deductible for Parts A or B. There will be copays and coinsurance.

In the Metro Denver, Colorado, area, we have eight Medicare Advantage plans for 2022. Lots of choices! Of course, if you live in another state or another area in Colorado, your plans may be different.

Here is a mockup of a normal Summary of Benefits for Healthcare and Drugs. This is not from an existing plan, but very close to what you will see with an actual MA HMO plan. Then we will look at how to interpret the costs and services.

BENEFITS	YOUR COST
Monthly Premium	*$0*
Doctor's Office Visit	*$0 for Primary/ $35 for Specialist*
Preventative Services	*$0*
Inpatient Hospital Care	*$275 per day: for days 1–5* *$0 copay per unlimited days after that*
Skilled Nursing Facility – SNF	*$0 copay per day: days 1–20* *$160 copay per day: days 21–48* *$0 copay per day: days 49–100*
Outpatient Surgery	*$250 copay* *Cost sharing for additional plan covered services will apply*
Diabetes Monitoring Supplies	*$0 copay*
Home Health Care	*$0 copay*
Diagnostic Radiology services (such as MRIs and CAT scans	*20% coinsurance*
Diagnostic test and procedures (Non-radiological)	*20% coinsurance or copay*
Lab Services	*$0 copay*
Outpatient X-rays	*$10 copay*
Ambulance	*$250 ground*
Emergency Care	*$90 copay (worldwide)*
Urgent Care	*$40 copay ($80 for worldwide services)*

| Annual out-of-pocket maximum | $4900 |

ADDITIONAL BENEFITS

Routine Physical	*$0 copay – one yearly*
Vision-routine eye exam	*$20 copay – one yearly*
Vision-eyewear	*$200 yearly allowance for eyeglasses, frames or contacts*
Hearing-routine exam	*$10 copay – one yearly*
Hearing aids	*$650 basic per ear/ $950 plus per ear/ 2 per year*
Silver Sneakers Fitness	*Basic membership at a Silver Sneakers network location*
Caregiver Solutions	*$0 copay – 24/7 help from a care manager*
Foot care	*$40 copay for routine foot care*
Nurse line	*24-hour RN availability*
Dental	*$1500 yearly*

DRUGS	DRUG TIERS	
Yearly Deductible	*$0 for Tiers 1 and 2*	*$480 for Tiers 3,4, and 5*
Initial Coverage	*Standard Retail*	*Preferred Mail Order*
Tier 1: Preferred Generic	*$0 copay*	*$0 copay*
Tier 2: Generic	*$4 copay*	*$12 copay*
Tier 3: Preferred Brand	*$47 copay*	*$135 copay*
Tier 4: Non-Preferred Drugs	*$100 copay*	*$300 copay*
Tier 5: Specialty Drugs	*29%*	*29%*

HOW TO READ THE SUMMARY

Here are a few things that are important when choosing a plan:

Premium: Our example has no premium.

Healthcare Deductible: Our example has no deductible for A or B.

Max Out-of-Pocket (MAX OOP): This can vary, but Medicare caps the MAX OOP at $7750. This is your safety net so if you have a year with numerous expenses, you will pay no more than the MAX OOP.

Copays and Coinsurance: Copays are fixed amounts you pay at the point of service, such as a copay for a doctor visit.

Coinsurance is a percentage of a charge. Most testing and scans have a 20% coinsurance.

Network: For HMOs you want to make sure your providers are in the network.

Part D: If you choose an MA plan with no Part D, disregard that table.

MA PREFERRED PROVIDER ORGANIZATIONS (PPO)

As with an HMO, a PPO has a network. But a couple of differences set a PPO apart. No referral is needed to see an in-network provider. And if you want to go out of the network for a service, you can, although you usually pay more. For example, you will pay 40% of the total cost for out-of-network doctor visits, hospital stays, and outpatient surgeries. A few PPOs allow you to use plan providers anywhere in the United States.

Benefits are very similar to those of an HMO. Monthly premiums for PPOs range from $0 to $60, but that varies from region to region and state to state.

PPOs were not meant for high-level usage because of cost, but for certain services, you may find it advantageous to see an occasional provider you like who is out of network. This can be handy when you are traveling out of network.

MA DRUG COVERAGE (MAPD)

Most MAs include Part D prescription drug coverage. These plans are designated MAPD. As your total drug costs rise, you move through three payment stages with different deductibles and copays: Initial Coverage, Coverage Gap, and Catastrophic.

Initial Coverage: You are in the Initial Coverage stage until your total drug costs reach $4430. These include your deductible of $480 or less (MAPD plans usually lower this), copays, and what your plan pays.

Coverage Gap: After your drug costs reach $4430, you are in the Coverage Gap. You will now pay 25% of drug costs until your True Out-of-Pocket Cost (TROOP) reaches $7050. To calculate TROOP, add your 25% of a drug's price to the 70% manufacturer's discount and you have 95%. If the price is $100, then $95 goes toward your $6350 limit.

Catastrophic Stage: After your drug costs reach $7050, you enter the Catastrophic Stage (unfortunate choice of terms!). Ironically, things get less expensive now. You will pay $3.95 for all generics that retail for under $72 and 5% for those over. For brand name drugs, you pay $9.85 for those under a $179 retail price and 5% for those over.

We do a drug cost analysis with all our clients. If you are taking several generic or branded drugs, a yearly analysis could save you money. Go to *www.medicare.gov* and click on Drug Coverage. We will show you where to find instructions for determining drug costs in Chapter 7.

MA PRIVATE FEE-FOR-SERVICE PLANS (PFFS)

Private Fee-for-Service Plans are unique because they have no network. You can use any Medicare-approved doctor who accepts the plan's payment schedule. For each appointment or service though, you must call the provider, let them know what plan you have, and ascertain that the provider will accept the plan's payment. You do not need referrals or a primary care physician. PFFS plans may or may not include Part D. If not, you can enroll in a standalone Part D plan.

We will see fewer of these plans in the future, as Medicare is pressuring MA carriers to use their network whenever possible.

MA SPECIAL NEEDS PLANS (SNP)

Special Needs Plans serve people with specific needs in three general areas:

C-SNP: C-SNP is for beneficiaries who have chronic or disabling conditions and require a prescribed care management program. Conditions include cardiovascular disease, diabetes, osteoarthritis, ESRD, HIV/AIDS, and mental disorders. A doctor must verify the enrollee's condition, and periodic proof is required that he or she continues to meet the C-SNP criteria. It's best to call Medicare at 800-633-4227 and make sure you follow all the guidelines.

I-SNP: I-SNP applies to those who are eligible for institutional care or care in long-term care institutions for at least 90 days. This can be a nursing home or an intermediate care facility such as one for the intellectually disabled.

D-SNP: D-SNP is for people who are dual-eligible for both Medicaid and Medicare.

All SNP plans include Part D plans. They also include networks and, in many cases, a much higher level of care and care management than other MA plans. Out-of-pocket costs can be eliminated or greatly reduced with SNP plans.

Those who qualify will have a flexible Special Enrollment Period (SEP).

COST PLANS

Cost plans are hybrids that offer the best parts of both MA plans and SUPPs. They are being phased out due to CMS requirements. As of 2019, they have been eliminated from counties with two or more competing MA plans. If you live in a county with fewer than two competing MA plans, you might be able to keep your Cost plan.

MA MEDICAL SAVINGS ACCOUNTS (MSA)

Medicare Savings Accounts combine a high-deductible MA plan with a personal savings account that is used to pay for healthcare expenses until the deductible is met. These plans have no Part D, so participants need to get a standalone drug plan.

MEDICARE ADVANTAGE PLANS ARE CHANGING

Changes come gradually with Medicare plans and vary from region to region and plan to plan. Here are a few changes being included in MA benefits going forward:

NO THERAPY CAP

In the past the number of visits for physical, speech, or occupational therapy was capped. No more. Congress permanently repealed the visit cap in exchange for a monetary cap of $2150 in 2022. If your total therapy costs reach that amount, Medicare requires your provider to confirm that your therapy is medically necessary before the limit can be raised.

TELEMEDICINE

Telemedicine is an exciting new development in healthcare. MA plans are expanding this area to cover mental health virtual visits and services to patients with end-stage renal disease or stroke.

CAREGIVER SOLUTIONS

Caregivers can now speak with a care manager who assists with resources on behalf of a loved one. MA plans can also pay for home health aides to help with daily living activities including eating, dressing, and personal care.

LIFESTYLE HELP

If a medical provider recommends benefits, they can be included in an MA. Home safety improvements such as grab bars and wheelchair ramps can be covered. Meals delivered to the home and transportation to doctor appointments can also qualify.

TIPS FROM PROFESSOR MEDICARE

Every fall before the Annual Enrollment Period begins on October 15, you will probably start receiving mailers from insurance carriers pitching a specific plan or menu of plans. This is the time of year when insurance companies ramp up their marketing and spending via tv, radio, internet, mail, and even telephone. It is against CMS policy for anyone outside your plan carrier or agent to call you regarding MA promotions. If you get those calls, report them to Medicare at 800-633-4227.

Be wary of agents who represent only one company or one plan. Called "captive agents," they will not be able to give you choices. As brokers, we represent eight MA insurance carriers, and most have multiple plans. When sitting with a client, we ask questions, listen carefully, and find the plan that fits that individual's needs. If we represented only one company, there is no way we could feel confident of finding the best fit.

Make sure your providers are in-network for the plan you are about to choose. Also, make sure your medications are covered and determine the yearly cost of those meds. Formularies change from plan to plan and you would be surprised to see the cost differences in medications. Be sure you are getting a plan that covers your medications with competitive pricing.

Have an idea of how much travel you will engage in. Will you stay in another state for months at a time? Will you travel cross-country in your RV? This is important because if your MA plan has no provisions for a national network, and few do, then you will be out of network if you are out of your area or state. If you have a PPO, you will have coverage but pay much more. With an HMO, you will have emergency and urgent care coverage, but nothing else. If you travel a lot, maybe it's better to look at a SUPP that allows you to use any provider in the United States who takes Medicare.

If you enroll in an MA plan during AEP from October 15–December 7, then change your mind, you can do so during the Open Enrollment Period (OEP) from January 1–March 31. You can change to another MA plan or go back to Original Medicare during OEP.

SUMMARY

Medicare Advantage plans are expanding benefits every year. For many people who have minimal healthcare needs, they are a good match. If your Part B premium is $170.10 a month and your MAPD plan, with Part D and no deductibles, has a $0 premium, you are getting broad coverage at a rate much lower than what you probably paid for under-65 insurance.

With a MAX OOP that must be $7550 or less, you also have a safety net so one bad year won't deplete your retirement savings.

Additional benefits such as fitness membership, vision, dental or hearing coverage, over-the-counter products and more add to a plan's appeal.

A wide variety of MA plans including HMOs, PPOs, PFFSs, SNPs, Cost plans, and MSPs allows you to find just the right coverage for your needs. We can help you sort through the plans.

CHAPTER QUESTIONS

1. When is the Annual Enrollment Period?
2. Do you need a referral if you have a PPO?
3. When do companies communicate their Annual Notice of Changes?
4. When is OEP and what can you do at that time?
5. Do you need a primary care physician with an HMO?

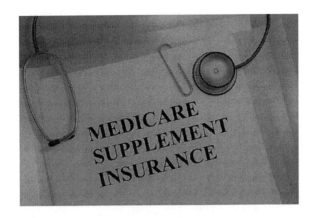

CHAPTER 5

MEDICARE SUPPLEMENT PLANS (SUPPS)

Marjorie has psoriatic arthritis, an auto-immune disease with no cure. She gets expensive injections in her doctor's office six times a year. Under her current employer plan, each costs her hundreds of dollars out of pocket. Routine tests add more expenses as she carefully monitors her condition. Marjorie wants to see a specialist in Phoenix who is one of the country's authorities on arthritis.

Which plan will best help Marjorie obtain the services she needs while containing costs? After a yearly deductible and monthly premium, a SUPP would reduce Marjorie's out of pocket to $0 while allowing her to obtain care from any Medicare provider[8] in any state.

Also called Medigap policies, SUPPs are sold by private health insurance companies to pay medical expenses not covered by Original Medicare, including deductibles, coinsurance, and copays. If you have frequent doctor visits, lab tests, or hospitalizations, **or** if you need an expensive surgery or long-term hospital stay, **or** if you need to see providers beyond your normal area, a SUPP may be the perfect choice for you to maximize care while containing costs.

In this chapter, we'll tell you everything you need to know about SUPPs including how they work, how much they cost, and how you can enroll or change plans.

HOW SUPPS WORK

When you use a service or provider who accepts Medicare, their office verifies that it covers the service. The provider bills Medicare, which pays the contracted amount, a percentage of the accepted charge. If Medicare pays 80% of a charge, then the 20% balance is electronically sent to your SUPP carrier, which pays your portion. All SUPPs follow this protocol. It's simple and clean. You won't need to hassle with payments, as your SUPP takes care of them.

Here is how a normal office visit works with a SUPP. Let's assume you have a Plan G. You see the dermatologist of your choice and show your Medicare and SUPP cards. Medicare pays 80% of the fee for services, leaving 20% for you to pay. But after

---

[8] A provider who accepts Medicare assignment and either accepts Medicare's payment as the full fee or charges the patient an excess charge over what Medicare allows.

your $233 yearly deductible, your SUPP picks up this 20%, covering the gap between what Medicare pays and the full-service charge. You have eliminated copays and coinsurance. If you have a Plan F, there is no yearly deductible.

This differs from how an MA plan works. With MA, you would go to a dermatologist in your network and have a copay from $0 to $50 in most cases. Or if you had outpatient surgery with an MAPD, you would pay the fixed rate of $140–$325. With a SUPP you would pay $0.

A MENU OF SUPP PLANS

Let's dig in. A wide variety of private insurance companies offer SUPPs. In our 80301 zip code, more than 35 companies will offer plans A, B, D, high-deductible F or G, F, G, K, L, M, and N for 2020. Do you see why we call it alphabet soup? Who was the knucklehead who named Medicare Parts A, B, C, and D, and then used the same alphabet to name plans? It's an area of constant confusion. But we digress.

Through a collaboration between CMS and the National Association of Insurance Commissioners, each state approves a slate of SUPPs whose healthcare benefits are identical. Plans with the same letter offer the same basic benefits, regardless of the carrier. That means all Plan Gs are the same no matter who you buy them from.

The only variable is the premium an insurance carrier charges. Some plans offer discounts that can lower the premium. Others offer services beyond the basic required coverage. For example, a few plans offer Silver Sneakers fitness programs as an added benefit.

	A	B	D	G*	K	L	M	N
Medicare Part A Coinsurance and hospital costs (up to an additional 365 days after Medicare benefits are used)	100%	100%	100%	100%	100%	100%	100%	100%
Medicare Part B coinsurance or copayment	100%	100%	100%	100%	50%	75%	100%	100%*
Blood (first 3 pints)	100%	100%	100%	100%	50%	75%	100%	100%
Part A hospice care coinsurance or copayment	100%	100%	100%	100%	50%	75%	100%	100%
Skilled nursing facility care coinsurance			100%	100%	50%	75%	100%	100%
Part A deductible		100%	100%	100%	50%	75%	50%	100%
Part B deductible								
Part B excess charges				100%				
Foreign travel emergency			80%	80%			80%	80%
Out-of-pocket limit					$6620	$3310		

- *Plan G offers a high-deductible plan in some states. You pay all Medicare costs (coinsurance, copayments, and deductibles) up to the deductible of $2370 (2021) before your policy pays anything.*
- *Plan N pays 100% of Part B coinsurance except for a $20 copayment for some office visits plus up to a $50 copayment for emergency room visits that are not followed by inpatient admission.*
- *For Plan K and Plan L, after meeting your yearly out-of-pocket limit and Part B deductible, the plan pays 100% of covered services for the rest of the calendar year.*
- *Foreign travel emergencies have a $250 deductible and 20% coinsurance up to a $50,000 maximum.*
- *A blank box in the chart indicates no coverage for that benefit.*

CASE STUDY MARJORIE

Remember Marjorie, the woman with psoriatic arthritis whom we profiled at the beginning of the chapter? It turned out that Plan G was perfect for her.

With MA plans Marjorie realized that she would have a 20% coinsurance for each injection, copays to see her specialist regularly, and coinsurance for her tests. With a Plan G SUPP, once she pays her $233 Part B deductible, she has no more copays or coinsurance for the injections, visits, or tests. She can schedule an appointment with the specialist in Phoenix who takes Medicare. Her premium for Plan G is around $110 per month.

IF YOU DON'T SEE YOUR PLAN ON THE CHART

Beginning in 2020 plans were not be allowed to waive the Part B deductible. Thus Plans C and F could no longer be sold to anyone who turned 65 after January 1, 2020. However, current subscribers may be grandfathered to keep their plans and those with eligibility before 2020 may still be able to purchase them. Many of our clients are enrolled in these plans:

Benefits	C	F
Medicare Part A Coinsurance and hospital costs (up to an additional 365 days after Medicare benefits are used)	100%	100%
Medicare Part B coinsurance or copayment	100%	100%
Blood (first 3 pints)	100%	100%
Part A hospice care coinsurance or copayment	100%	100%
Skilled nursing facility care coinsurance	100%	100%
Part A deductible	100%	100%
Part B deductible	100%	100%
Part B excess charges	100%	100%
Foreign travel emergency	80%	80%
Out-of-pocket limit		

In 2010 Plans H, I, and J were discontinued since SUPP plans no longer cover Part D drug benefits. Plan E was removed in 1988.

Massachusetts, Minnesota, and Wisconsin have SUPP plans that are standardized differently from these listings. For more information on those plans, download the CMS publication Choosing a Medigap Policy: A Guide to Health Insurance for People with Medicare *from our site:* www.ProfessorMedicare.com/.

HOW TO CHOOSE A SUPP PLAN

SUPP plans have evolved to provide more choices in coverage and costs. For example, Plan B covers 100% of hospital coinsurance while Plan L pays only 50%. Of course, Plan B's premium is higher than Plan L's. With nine SUPP plans slated for 2022, how do you compare the plans to decide which is right for you?

When choosing a SUPP here are key factors to consider:

- Monthly premium
- Financial rating
- History of rate increases
- Average yearly increase because of age
- Discounts
- Plan benefits

When we meet with clients who have decided they want a SUPP and not an MA plan, it's because they want one or all the following:

- Can use any provider who takes Medicare
- Are not restricted by a network or geographic boundary
- Want to be free of copays and coinsurance
- No need for a referral
- No MAX OOP to deal with

Over the years we have mostly recommended Plans F, G, and N. Traditionally, Plan F has been the #1 choice for SUPPs, as it offers the most comprehensive benefits (but also the highest premium). Plan F dispenses with the Part B deductible and pays 100% for Medicare-approved services. However as of 2020, Plan F is no longer available to new Medicare subscribers.

No worries! We have found that Plan G is a smarter choice anyway. Plan G is exactly like Plan F with one exception—with Plan G there is a once-yearly Part B deductible of $233. After that your copays and coinsurance are eliminated. The lower premium ($20–$30 less than Plan F) will more than offset the deductible. Plus, Plan G protects you from excess charges by providers. Both Donna and I got Plan G years ago because of the savings.

Are you interested in economy or luxury? Plan N is a Volkswagen Beetle compared to Plan G's Cadillac. Plan N's premium is about 20% less than Plan G's. You still pay the Part B deductible, $20 per office visit, and $50 for the ER. It does not cover excess charges.

You must assess whether the premium savings offsets what you would pay for office visits and the ER. We have many clients who see providers only three to five times a year, so Plan N works well for them.

It would be helpful if the letter plans were ranked according to a cost/benefit analysis—you know, platinum, gold, silver, etc. But they are not. As we do price comparisons, we see plans like Plan B and Plan D with fewer covered benefits but premiums just about level with Plan G. It makes no sense to enroll you in a plan with fewer benefits and more cost.

CASE STUDY ED AND LOIS

Ed and Lois are newly retired. He turns 65 in March and Lois will in May. They plan to sell their home, rent a small apartment for six to eight months a year, and then travel in their RV for the remaining months. Both are healthy and each takes two generic medications. They are active bicyclists and eat a healthy diet. Before Medicare they never met the deductible in their ACA plan and saw doctors about a half dozen times a year.

We showed them MA plans and SUPPs. Because of their minimal use of their past plans, they leaned toward an MA plan with no premium.

But when we talked about travel and being out of network while on the road, they understood that choosing a SUPP with national coverage and no network was their realistic choice. Since their usage was so minimal, Plan N worked well, and their premiums were around $90 a month.

This was in 2018. For 2022 we will have an MA PPO plan that they can use nationwide. We will call Ed and Lois and let them know they have a great new choice!

FOREIGN TRAVEL EMERGENCY COVERAGE

Four SUPPS—Plans D, G, M, and N—have foreign travel coverage. After a $250 deductible, you pay 20% of services up to a lifetime maximum of $50,000.

We always advise our clients to add some travel insurance. It's inexpensive and has emergency coverage with no coinsurance or copay. It avoids the SUPP deductible and 20% coinsurance. Check with us for travel insurance coverage.

SUPP PREMIUMS

If all Plan Gs are the same, why do three companies charge different premiums for it? Insurance companies use three methods to describe SUPPs and determine premium payments:

Age-Attained Pricing: A carrier bases your premium on your age when they issue your policy. The premium increases as you age.

Issue-Aged Pricing: A carrier bases the premium on your age when they issue your policy, and premiums increase when the company has a "statewide increase." They say there is no increase due to age.

Community-Rated Pricing: Carriers charge the same premium to all beneficiaries regardless of their age or overall health. Increases can be due to inflation, carrier expenses, etc.

These rating methods seem more related to marketing and sales than transparency. Before you buy a plan, check out the carrier's history of increases.

However, the past is no guarantee of future premiums. Sometimes clients ask whether rates seem to increase faster with certain plans. For example, will your rates go up more with Plan B or Plan G?

Plans with fewer young enrollees tend to increase rates more. This is because older Medicare recipients make more claims than younger ones. When a plan becomes heavy with older beneficiaries, it lacks enough younger subscribers to offset the higher incidence of claims.

Every carrier has occasional across-the-board increases and increases due to your age. They may describe the increase as caused by inflation or expenses or claims, but the fact is, you will pay more as you age. You can't get around it.

Go with a solid company and compare premiums with other carriers. In Colorado we see yearly SUPP premium increases because of age. Plans also institute across-the-board increases from time to time. As brokers, we check a carrier's history of increases and the current rate to make sure a client is getting a competitive premium.

WHEN TO ENROLL IN A SUPP

OPEN ENROLLMENT PERIOD (OEP)

When you first enroll in Medicare Parts A and B and it begins on the first day of your birth month, you will have six months to enroll in a SUPP. During this OEP you can choose any SUPP offered in your area.

Safeguards ensure that you will not be denied coverage:

- You can't be denied coverage for health reasons.
- You can't be charged more for health reasons.
- A company cannot delay your coverage.

EXCEPTIONS

If you have a pre-existing condition that has been treated or diagnosed within six months before your SUPP starts and you have not had "creditable"[9] coverage, you may choose to pay for

---

[9] Creditable health care coverage means you participated in an approved group, individual, student, children's, or government plan.

services. Although Original Medicare will cover the condition, your SUPP may not and you would have copays or coinsurance. Your other option is to wait six months for full coverage to begin.

If you have had creditable coverage from any other health plan six months before applying for a SUPP, you will be covered with no extra charges.

Plans that are not part of the ACA or a major medical plan with an employer may not be creditable. These are known as "junk" plans. Call the State Health Insurance Assistance Program (SHIP) in your state to verify coverage.

If you have a Guaranteed Issue (GI) right (see below), there is no waiting period for pre-existing conditions.

OVER 65 AND MOVING OFF AN EMPLOYER PLAN

After ending an employer healthcare plan, you have eight months to enroll in Part B and then the OEP for a SUPP lasts six months.

GUARANTEED ISSUE (GI)

Even if you are not in an OEP for a SUPP, certain situations require that you be guaranteed coverage:

Guaranteed Issue if...	You can buy...	When?
Your MA plan leaves the area or stops care,	A, B, G, K or L sold in your state	60 days before your MA ends or 63 days after it ends

or you move out of your service area		
You have Original Medicare and an employer plan or Cobra, and the plan is ending	A, B, G, K or L If you have Cobra, you can get a SUPP or wait till Cobra ends	63 days after the latest of: the coverage ending, a notice the coverage is ending, or the date on a claim denial
You have Original Medicare plus a Select Policy and move out of the area	A, B, G, K or L sold in your state	60 days before Select coverage ends – no later than 63 days after it ends
You join an MA or PACE plan when first eligible for Part A at 65 and within the first year want to switch to Original Medicare	Any SUPP sold by any carrier in your state	60 days before your MA coverage ends – no later than 63 days after it ends – rights may be extended under certain conditions
You dropped a SUPP to join an MA plan or switched to a Select plan for the 1st time and you want to go back to the SUPP	You must go back to the same SUPP and same carrier you had before switching. If it's not available, go to A, B, G, K or L	60 days before your MA coverage ends – no later than 63 days after it ends – rights may be extended under certain conditions
Your SUPP ends or goes bankrupt	A, B, G, K or L sold in your state	No later than 63 days from the date coverage ends

You leave an MA plan or drop a SUPP because the carrier misled you or broke rules	A, B, G, K or L sold in your state	No later than 63 days from the date coverage ends

Guaranteed Issue rights dictate that insurance carriers must:

- Sell you a policy
- Cover pre-existing conditions
- Not charge you more because of your health

WHAT IF YOU WANT TO CHANGE YOUR SUPP?

There is no AEP for SUPPs. That means if you want to move from one plan to another or from one carrier to another, you can do it at any time. After your six-month open enrollment though, you will have to answer health questions and can be denied coverage if your answers don't pass the company's underwriting requirements. As brokers we have a good sense of what can pass and what can't.

I have had a few clients whose SUPPs had a small rate increase of less than $10 a month. Nervous, they wanted to change plans. But once you change to another company, what is to say their rates won't rise? All carriers have rate increases. When? We don't know until they happen. Unless a company has big increases year after year, it's best to stay with what you have.

FINANCIAL RATINGS

You don't need to worry that you might jeopardize your coverage by enrolling in a SUPP with unscrupulous or incompetent management. Insurance company financial ratings are graded by A.M. Best and S&P. Only one company in my area has a B. The rest are B+ to A+. States will not approve plans with low financial ratings, so don't be too concerned. If yours is at least a B+, it's solid.

You also have ample protection against a company shutting down. Let's say you enrolled in a SUPP with Company ABC and that company went bankrupt. Medicare guarantees that you can enroll in another SUPP with no underwriting or health questions.

WHICH PROVIDERS TAKE SUPPS?

How do you find providers who take SUPPs? Easy! If a provider takes Parts A and B, then they must take your SUPP. The term that tells you a provider accepts Medicare is "accepts Medicare assignment." That means they have agreed to accept payment from Medicare.

Here is how to find providers:

1. Go to *www.medicare.gov.*
2. From the menu bar at the top, click "Find doctors and other health professionals."
3. Enter your city or zip code on the left and your target on the right. You can use filters for mileage and other search parameters.
4. Once you find the doctor, facility, or group, you need to locate this phrase: "Accepts Medicare-approved payment amounts."

If they accept approved payments, you can use your SUPP with that provider. If they do not accept payment, call their office to verify their status regarding accepting Medicare.

YOUR MEDICARE SUMMARY NOTICE (MSN)

I hesitated before deciding to include this section on billing and reports. After considering how many questions we get from clients on the topic, we are diving into it.

The Medicare Summary Notice is not a bill. We get calls from clients who are upset when they get their summaries in the mail and see large numbers associated with services. If there is a bill, you will get it from your provider, not from Medicare or your SUPP.

If you have received Part A or B services for a three-month period, you will get an MSN. It shows:

- All your services or supplies that providers and suppliers billed to Medicare during the three-month period
- What Medicare paid
- The maximum amount you may owe the provider
- How much you have paid toward your $233 Part B deductible

If you don't use any services or medical supplies during that three-month period, you won't get a summary for that period.

If you owe money for services, your provider's office will bill you.

AARP has a page that helps you decode the MSN: *https://www.aarp.org/health/medicare-insurance/info-05-2011/popup-part-b-medicare-summary-notice.html#inline20*.

If you haven't done so, go to *www.mymedicare.gov* and create an account. You will need your Medicare claim number to do this.

Why? This is where you can track claims, plans and coverages, and providers and services. You can also sign up to have your quarterly Medicare Summary Notice emailed to you. This will save you time and effort as you use your plan.

MAXIMUM YOU MAY BE BILLED

If Medicare approved your service, you may see an amount on your MSN under the heading "Maximum You May Be Billed." You may or may not receive a bill from the provider. I see this a lot on my summaries but have not received a bill for anything for years. I had a few chiropractic visits this year and my MSN detailed each visit as follows:

Total Amount Charged:	$49.00
Medicare Approved:	$27.62
Medicare Paid Provider:	$21.66
Total Amount You May be Charged:	$5.52

That was a normal summary explanation. Instead of reacting, I waited to see if the provider would bill me. He did not.

SERVICES NOT COVERED

Important! Check your summary. If you see a note that services are not covered, that means Medicare will not pay nor will your SUPP. SUPPs only pay after Medicare approves a service and pays its share.

Call the provider's billing office to see if they used the correct code for billing and that the service was deemed "medically necessary."

If you find that the billing was correct, and you are not satisfied, you can file an appeal. Each MSN has an appeal form and instructions.

SUMMARY

Medicare Supplement Plans are a great way to protect yourself financially if you have a chronic medical condition, need expensive surgery or long-term hospitalization, or want to use a provider outside your geographic area. With nine SUPP plans to choose from, each with its own benefits and costs, there is a plan to fit everyone's needs.

Now you know what to look for so you can make the right choice. You know how to interpret your summary of benefits. And you know when you can enroll or change your SUPP should your situation change.

CHAPTER QUESTIONS

1. Will Plan F be sold in 2022?

2. What is Issue-Aged pricing?

3. Will your Supplement premium stay the same?

4. Can a company raise your premium if you have too many claims?

5. Do Supplements include drug coverage?

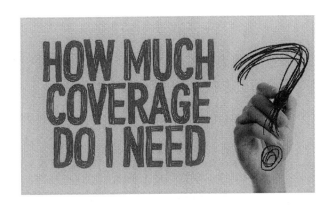

CHAPTER 6

CHOICES, CHOICES . . .

MEDICARE ADVANTAGE OR MEDICARE SUPPLEMENT?

When we began the book, we listed four questions we address when working with clients. Here they are again:

1. When do I enroll in Medicare?
2. Should I stay with Original Medicare only and add a Part D plan? At what cost?
3. Should I enroll in a Medicare Advantage plan with or without Part D drug coverage? At what cost?
4. Should I stay with Original Medicare and add a Medigap/Supplement plan and Part D plan? At what cost?

Chapter 8 will provide all you need to answer the first question. After you enroll in Parts A and B, you can choose your coverage package.

Which of options 2–4 is best for you? Obviously, you want a plan that will provide the best coverage at the lowest cost. You want it to cover your specific situation and not include features you don't need.

To determine whether to enroll in an MA plan or a SUPP, you'll need to look at the type and cost of healthcare services you require, how frequently you will use them, what providers you prefer, and what out-of-pocket costs you are comfortable with.

MA PLANS VS. SUPPS

SUPPS are like a prix fixe meal at a restaurant—everything is included for a set price. MAs are like ordering à la carte—you pay for each item separately.

Replacing Original Medicare, an MA plan offers the same services as Parts A and B but may add coverage for vision, hearing, dental, and/or fitness. Many also include Part D drug coverage. The low cost of MAs appeals to individuals who need infrequent medical care.

An MA HMO is the more restrictive, requiring you to get referrals and use network providers. But most plans balance that with no premium and no deductible for Parts A and B.

An MA PPO requires no referrals. Its network is similar to that of an HMO, but you may elect to pay extra for out-of-network care. PPOs may charge premiums and all have copays.

SUPPs appeal to people who need frequent or expensive healthcare, want the flexibility to see providers outside their geographic area, and/or hate the surprise of mounting costs from copays and coinsurance. SUPPs do what their name suggests—they are add-ons that supplement Parts A and B. They come with a premium, but reduce or eliminate out-of-pocket costs. Most SUPPs are free of copays, coinsurance, and referrals. Plan G for 2022 carries a yearly $233 deductible,[10] but after that you pay $0 for care. Part D must be purchased separately. With no network, subscribers may obtain care from any U.S. Medicare provider.

As with MAs, there are multiple SUPP options, varying in coverage and price.

CASE STUDY STEVE

Our discussion with Steve helped him decide which health plan variables were important to him. He gave us all we needed to make the best recommendation.

Steve is skeptical about the healthcare system. He doesn't trust doctors and avoids them. His wife died four years ago from lung cancer and it was a slow, painful process for them both. The only thing he liked was the kind treatment she received in the hospice. Steve has ample financial resources so money for premiums isn't an issue. Fit and healthy, he is an avid bicyclist who competes in events in the Southwest, traveling three months a year.

We looked at an MA plan, but Steve didn't want to deal with a network. He liked the freedom to choose any doctor who takes Medicare anywhere in the United States. As soon as we learned how averse Steve was to a network, we stopped proposing any MA plan and showed him a SUPP. Because of his travel and risk of a riding injury, Steve decided a Plan G SUPP would work best.

---

[10] Older Plans C and F have no deductible, but as of 2020 no new plans will be sold. Current subscribers may be grandfathered.

He also liked a low-priced Part D plan that covered his two generic medications.

A FINANCIAL COMPARISON

Let's look at the major financial distinctions between MA plans and SUPPs. In the following chart, you can easily see which plans have deductibles, networks, and extra benefits:

Premium	*MA Plans* *Most have zero*	*SUPPS* *Yes- vary with plan*
Deductible	*Most have zero*	*Plan B is $233 with most. Some have Part A deductible*
Max Out of Pocket	*$7550 is maximum. Most have less*	*Only 2 have MAX OOP*
Network	*Yes*	*No*
Access to providers	*Area specific*	*Anywhere in US*
Copays and coinsurance	*Yes*	*Most have zero*
Include Part D	*Yes- with a few exceptions*	*No*
Referral needed	*Yes, for most HMO – no for PPO*	*No*
Premium Rate Increases	*rare*	*Yearly*
Extra benefits- fitness, dental, hearing, vision and more	*Most do*	*Only Fitness with a few plans*

Next, we offer a direct comparison between an MA plan and a SUPP. Using numbers similar to plans in our area gives a close approximation of what you would find in this marketplace. If you live in another state's metropolitan area, the numbers should be close to what you see here. For the SUPP, we are using Plan G for a 65-year-old female. G is our go-to plan as a replacement for Plan F. You will see monthly and yearly numbers. We are using an HMO for the MA choice.

CATEGORIES	MA	SUPP
Part A Deductible	$0	$0/ Some have Part A deductible*
Part B Deductible	$0	Plan B is $233 with most.
Max Out of Pocket	$7550 is maximum. Most have less	Only 2 have MAX OOP
Part D Deductible	TBD**	TBD**
Part D Premium	$0	$32 average
Part B Premium	$170.10	$170.10
Plan Premium	$0 for most	$110 for Plan G female
Monthly Cost	$170.10	$312.10
Yearly Cost	$2041.20	$3978.20

*Some SUPPs have a full or partial Part A deductible. Most MA plans have no deductible, but some do. Original Medicare always has a deductible.

**The Part D Deductible for 2022 is $480, but it varies from plan to plan. Some plans have no deductible. Others may charge an amount less than $480, and some charge a deductible for certain drug tiers. Check your plan for an exact number.

CASE STUDY LOUISE

For Louise, cost was a critical issue. We helped her compare plans and find the one that would provide the care she needed while keeping her costs in check.

Louise is turning 65 and has an ACA plan with a premium of around $400 a month after tax help. It has a $6000 deductible that she reached in June. Louise fell on her shoulder and needed an emergency room visit, surgery, about 20 rehab appointments, and medications.

She feels better but her pocketbook is crying. Her small retirement income requires her to work part time at Home Depot.

We verified that her providers were in-network for two of our local MA plans and showed her one with a $0 premium, drug plan, vision benefit, fitness benefit, and most important, $0 deductible. All Louise will pay is her Medicare Part B premium of $170.10 a month. Her copays and coinsurance are reasonable and much less than what she had before turning 65. Another happy camper.

HOW TO INTERPRET THE NUMBERS

Like Louise, lowering premium costs may be your primary consideration in choosing a plan. Or like Steve, a different variable may be the deciding factor. The charts and numbers above will help you compare costs.

What we did not include are copays and coinsurance because they vary so wildly from person to person. To approximate your out-of-pocket costs, look at what you spent last year. If your health is much the same as it was in 2021, you can make an educated guess for expenses. If you know you will have a surgery or procedure or have some future treatments to consider, put those into the equation.

Cost is only one factor. How about travel? Do you plan to be in your home area most of the year or will you live out of state for months? Are you ok with networks?

If you are looking at an MA plan, are you comfortable having a MAX OOP? Chances are small that you will ever reach it.

If you are leaning toward an MA plan, see which plan(s) your providers accept with the understanding that they can add or subtract accepted plans during the year.

These considerations result from our interactions with clients over the years and should help you in your process of choosing a plan.

CHANGING YOUR MA OR SUPP

The decision you make during your IEP or SEP is not permanent. Every year during the AEP you can move from one plan to another.

Medicare offers new enrollees a grace period in which to change coverage without answering medical questions. If you turn 65 and enroll in an MA plan, you have a year to move to a SUPP with no medical underwriting. If you are not 100% sure you'll like your new MA plan, you have a built-in exit strategy for year one.

If you are moving into a SUPP outside Medicare's grace period and do not have Guaranteed Issue rights, you will need to pass a company's medical underwriting. For MA plans, there are no health questions.

Even though your choice of a plan is not permanent, we want it to be your best choice. After showing clients the Medicare basics including parts and plans, we get a strong sign of which coverage will work best. Additional questions get the ball rolling and help us assess what you need and how your needs fit with what is available.

SUMMARY

Everyone wants great healthcare at a bargain price. Original Medicare is limited in what it covers, so companies created new plans to replace or supplement it. These Medical Advantage and Supplement plans offer subscribers a world of new choices in treatment coverage and cost management.

Although the number of plans and choices can seem daunting at first, whether to enroll in an MA plan or a SUPP boils down to 1) your health needs, 2) your preferences about networks, copays, referrals, and provider locations, and 3) costs.

Professor Medicare is happy to help you analyze your situation or discuss your choice to make sure your plan meets your needs and expectations.

CHAPTER QUESTIONS

1. Do I need to answer health questions to change my Medicare Advantage plan?
2. Do Supplements have a lot of extra benefits like Medicare Advantage plans?
3. Do most Medicare Advantage plans include a Part B deductible?
4. Can I get a Medicare Advantage plan without a network?
5. If I just had a heart attack and want to change my Supplement, would that be easy to do?

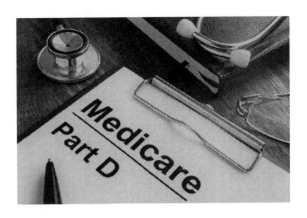

CHAPTER 7

PART D: DRUG COVERAGE

You probably saw media coverage of the skyrocketing price increases for the EpiPen epinephrine auto-injector. In 2007 a two-pack cost about $100. After a new company bought the drug rights, it gradually raised the price to $600, increasing its profits to $1.1 billion a year.[11]

---

[11] Beth Mole, "Years after Mylan's Epic EpiPen Price Hikes, it Finally Gets a Generic Rival," *Ars Technica,* August 17, 2018, https://arstechnica.com/science/2018/08/fda-approves-generic-version-of-mylans-600-epipens-but-the-price-is-tbd/.

Insulin cost about 75 cents per vial in the 1960s.[12] Today, although it only costs between $2–$6 to produce,[13] insulin is sold for about $275.[14] Prices tripled over the last 15 years.

Starting in 2021, Medicare Part D and Medicare Advantage Plans with Part D initiated a $35 cap on insulin copays. The cap is being applied to all coverage stages. This means beneficiaries will not have to negotiate deductibles or "donut hole" prices to get the $35 copay. That was wonderful news.

The newest drugs incite the worst sticker shock. A 24-week treatment for hepatitis C runs $150,000–$189,000.[15]

Increasingly, people ration or forego medications they can't afford. Having a prescription plan can mean the difference between sickness and health or even life and death. Fortunately for seniors, Medicare has a plan for that—Part D. An easy way to remember Part D is that **D = D**rugs.

Medicare began in 1965 but had no prescription drug coverage until 2006. Now Part D covers 73% of all Medicare enrollees— about 44 million Americans. It makes up around 13% of total Medicare payments to providers and suppliers. The average prescription cost per person varies and depends on the use of brand name as opposed to generic drugs.

[12] R. Scott Rappold, "Families Cross Borders in Search for Affordable Insulin," *WebMD,* July 18, 2019, https://www.webmd.com/diabetes/news/20190718/spiking-insulin-costs-put-patients-in-brutal-bind.

[13] Ed Silverman, "Insulin Prices Could Be Much Lower and Drug Makers Would Still Make Healthy Profits," *Business Insider,* September 26, 2018, https://www.businessinsider.com/insulin-prices-could-be-much-lower-and-drug-makers-would-still-make-healthy-profits-2018-9.

[14] Danielle K. Roberts, "The Deadly Costs of Insulin," *AJMC,* June 10, 2019, https://www.ajmc.com/contributor/danielle-roberts/2019/06/the-deadly-costs-of-insulin.

[15] Rachel Nall, "How Much Does Hepatitis C Treatment Cost?" *Medical News Today,* November 21, 2018, https://www.medicalnewstoday.com/articles/323767.php.

If you have Original Medicare, you can enroll in Part D. Many MAs include Part D coverage.

Of all the parts of Medicare, Part D is the most obtuse, confusing, and difficult to understand. But *Professor Medicare* is here to cut through the legalese so you understand your options. We will explain enrollment, plans, tiers, copays, the Donut Hole, and extra help. We will show you how to create a drug list at *Medicare.gov* so you can track your meds and their costs.

Take your time with this section.

Every year

Jan.	Feb.	Mar.	Apr.	May.	June	July	Aug.	Sept.	Oct.	Nov.	Dec

October 15 - December 7

ENROLLMENT

Remember your Initial Enrollment Period (IEP)? The same period applies to Parts A, B, C, and D. If you enroll in Part A and/or Part B, you can also enroll in a drug plan—however, you are not automatically enrolled in Part D.

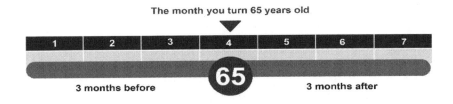

The month you turn 65 years old

| 1 | 2 | 3 | 4 | 5 | 6 | 7 |

65

3 months before   3 months after

During your IEP you must choose a standalone Part D plan or one included in an MA Plan. If you qualify for a Low-Income

Subsidy (LIS) or Medicaid, you may be auto-enrolled in a Part D plan. If you have an employer plan, your Part D enrollment period is shown in the chart above.

Medicare does not require you to enroll in a Part D plan. But if you do not enroll during your IEP and then later decide you want drug coverage, you may be subject to a permanent fine.[16] Medicare gives you 63 days from the last day of your IEP before the fines start.

What if you want to change plans or enroll for the first time? You may do that during the AEP.

PART D PLANS

Standalone Part D plans are sold to individuals who have Original Medicare, an MA Private Fee-for-Service (PFFS) plan, or a Medicare Savings Account (MSA). In our 80301 zip code, there are 26 plans with monthly premiums between $5.50–$113.20. Most of our members choose plans with premiums between $5.50–$32 a month.

The second type of Part D is included in an MA plan, and it's abbreviated MAPD. Not all plans have Part D.

That was simple enough. Now we will take a running leap into the wacky world of Part D and how it works.

OUT-OF-POCKET COSTS

Part D coverage does not mean your prescriptions are free. You will still have copays for drugs and must meet deductibles before

---

[16] For information on Part D fines, see Appendix E.

coverage kicks in. Let's look at what you'll pay when you get a prescription from the pharmacy.

DRUG TIERS

Brand name and generic drugs are categorized into five tiers according to their retail prices and how much of the cost you will share. As you move up the levels, drugs get more expensive and your share increases.

Each plan has its own formulary, a tiered list of both generic and brand name drugs that a committee of independent physicians and pharmacists has determined offer the greatest value. Formularies, including Medicare's, change yearly. Plans can drop drugs mid-year. Drugs can move from brand to generic or from Tier 2 to Tier 3. Nothing is permanently fixed in a tier or as a cost.

Here is a normal tier structure with some mock prices shown in the chart below. These are close to what you will see in your marketplace:[17]

- Tier 1: Low-cost generic drugs
- Tier 2: Preferred generics
- Tier 3: Preferred brand name drugs and non-preferred generics
- Tier 4: Non-preferred brand names and non-preferred generics
- Tier 5: High-cost brand name and generics that may require special permission or monitoring

---

[17] We used this chart in the section on MAPD plans.

Yearly Deductible	$0 for Tiers 1 and 2	$480 for Tiers 3,4, and 5
Initial Coverage	*Standard Retail*	*Preferred Mail Order*
Tier1: Preferred Generic	*$0 copays*	*$0 copay*
Tier2: Generic	*$4 copays*	*$12 copays*
Tier3: Preferred Brand	*$47 copays*	*$131 copays*
Tier4: Non-Preferred Drugs	*Coinsurance or copay*	*Coinsurance or copay*
Tier5: Specialty Drugs	*29%*	*29%*

In the chart a $480 deductible applies only for Tier 3 and up. That means you pay no deductible if all your meds are generic and in the first two tiers. Some plans offer lower prices at Preferred Pharmacy locations. Be sure to locate these and take advantage of those savings.

Getting your prescriptions through mail order can save you money, but not always. Mail order is very easy to start and simple to maintain. When you get your member card for your MAPD or Part D plan, call customer service and ask to set up mail order. My plan gave me a phone number for my provider to call, and after I gave my provider the number, his office took care of it— a very easy process. I get my generics every 90 days along with reminders for refills.

Now that you have seen the tiers and pricing, let's look at deductibles.

COVERAGE PERIODS

Part D recognizes four coverage periods. As your drug costs increase, you move from one period to the next. Each has its own spending levels, deductible, copays, and/or coinsurance. If your Part D coverage is part of an MA plan, please see Chapter 4 for details specific to your type of plan.

DEDUCTIBLE PERIOD

The Part D Deductible for 2022 is $480. That is standard for every drug plan. Until you meet your deductible, you will pay full price for medications. After you meet the deductible, your plan helps pay for the cost. Carriers may choose to lower the deductible, eliminate it, or only use it for certain tiers. Some plans have no deductible. So don't assume $480 is your deductible. Check your plan first.

INITIAL COVERAGE PERIOD

After you meet your deductible, you are in the Initial Coverage Period. You pay a copay or coinsurance portion of the total drug cost and your plan pays the rest. For example, if a med costs $32, you will pay $8 and your plan pays $24. That $32 cost accumulates toward your total drug cost. You will receive monthly statements from your plan and can track the costs.

COVERAGE GAP PERIOD (DONUT HOLE)

When your total drug costs (including the deductible) reach $4430 after January 1 of 2022, you enter the Donut Hole or Coverage Gap. When that happens, you will pay 25% of both generic and brand name drug costs. That amount plus what your plan and the brand name drug manufacturer pay go toward your true out-of-pocket costs (TROOP).

TROOP FOR BRAND NAME DRUGS

- Your 25% coinsurance for the brand name drug
- 70% paid by the drug manufacturer
- An additional 5% is paid by your Part D plan, but it is not included in TROOP

TROOP FOR GENERIC DRUGS

- Your 25% coinsurance for the generic drug
- No other amounts paid by the plan or manufacturer are part of TROOP

CATASTROPHIC COVERAGE

When your TROOP reaches $7050 for 2022, you are out of the Donut Hole and into Catastrophic Coverage (poor choice of words!). Ironically, things will get better for you financially as you finally get a break on costs. For example, if a generic med retails for less than $72, you pay $3.95. If it's over $72 retail, you pay 5%. For brands, it's $9.85 if less than $179 retail and 5% if over.

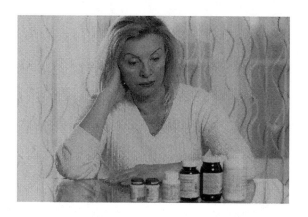

A TIP FROM PROFESSOR MEDICARE

If you take only one or two Tier 1 or Tier 2 meds, don't be concerned—you won't get near the Donut Hole. But if you have a few brand name medications, pay attention to your monthly statements. They will show when you are nearing the Coverage Gap, which will help you plan for expenses.

CHOOSING A PLAN

If the foregoing maelstrom of tiers, copays, Coverage Gaps, TROOP, and Catastrophic Coverage wasn't enough to send your brain in search of a lobotomy, now you need to make sense of them to choose a plan.

How do you decide which plan is best for you? When we meet with clients, we use the *Part D Plan Finder* at *www.Medicare.gov* (link to instructions:
https://www.medicare.gov/find-a-plan/staticpages/help-faq.aspx).

With MAPDs and standalone Part D plans, we can enter a client's medications and get a clear report on their expected drug costs.

The Plan Finder offers a deep analysis that covers the following:

- Cost for each drug
- Costs for a year
- Costs from current date to end of year
- Whether you will enter the Donut Hole
- Plan comparisons and much more

After you enter your medications into the Plan Finder, you will want to print your results to a PDF or to paper. There is no way to save the results online.

Since plans have different formularies and different costs, we use the *Medicare.gov* Plan Finder with all our clients who take medications. The health benefits in one MA Plan may be strong, but if its Part D costs are more than those in other MA plans, it may not be the wisest choice.

When you get your Annual Notice of Changes (ANOC) in September, be sure to read it carefully. Plans change yearly. Premiums go up and down. Formularies change. Standard and preferred pharmacies change. If you want to change plans, you have from October 15–December 7 to do so.

Fun stuff, eh?

COVERAGE RULES

Medicare and individual plan rules determine whether you must jump through extra hoops to be covered. These protect both your safety and the bottom line. It's good to familiarize yourself with these guidelines.

VACCINES

Both Part B and Part D cover vaccines.

Part B covers:

- Hepatitis B vaccine (for patients at high or intermediate risk)
- Influenza virus vaccine
- Pneumococcal pneumonia vaccine

- Vaccines directly related to treatment of an injury or direct exposure to a disease or condition

Part D covers (expect copays):

- Shingles (herpes zoster) vaccine
- Tdap (tetanus, diphtheria, and pertussis) vaccine
- MMR (measles, mumps, and rubella) vaccines
- BCG (bacille Calmette-Guerin) vaccine for tuberculosis
- Meningococcal vaccines
- Hepatitis A and Hepatitis B vaccines for low-risk beneficiaries
- Certain self-administered insulin shots

PRIOR AUTHORIZATION

Some drugs require prior authorization to ensure that they meet plan criteria. You may need to contact both the plan and your provider to manage this. If you don't meet all the requirements, your provider can appeal that the medication is medically necessary. If the request is approved, the plan will cover the drug.

STEP THERAPY

If your provider prescribes a brand name drug, the plan may ask that you try a less expensive generic first. If that doesn't give a satisfactory result, then you would be stepped up to the brand. If your provider requests an exemption, stating that it is medically necessary that you take the brand first, you may start with the more expensive medication. The provider can also request an exception if there is a chance the less expensive drug might cause an adverse health effect.

QUANTITY LIMITS

The plan may want to limit your intake of a drug due to safety or cost reasons. For example, if a drug is normally given once a day but your provider prescribes it twice a day for you, the plan may object. If your provider states it is necessary, the plan may grant an exception.

OPIOID SAFETY CHECKS

In 2016 prescription opioid overdoses led to more than 20,000 deaths in the United States. Among adults younger than 50, drug overdoses are the leading cause of death.[18]

Because of this, the dispensing of opioids has come under a microscope. If you take them, expect scrutiny. Expect reviews of your opioid prescriptions and limits on dosage and number of pills. Expect reviews of all your medications and how they interact with opioids. You may be enrolled in a drug management program with safety reviews and limitations on which pharmacies you may use.

---

[18] "Opioid Addiction," *Genetics Home Reference,* NIH U.S. National Library of Medicine, October 29, 2019, https://ghr.nlm.nih.gov/condition/opioid-addiction#statistics.

DO YOU NEED EXTRA HELP TO PAY FOR PART D?[19]

LOW-INCOME SUBSIDY (LIS)

The Low-Income Subsidy is a government program that helps people with low incomes pay Part D monthly premiums, annual deductibles, coinsurance, and copayments.

Dependent upon a beneficiary's income and resources, the subsidy averages $4900 per year. Being in the program eliminates the Part D Donut Hole or Coverage Gap and late enrollment fines.

ELIGIBILITY

You may qualify for the LIS available under Medicare Part D if your:

- Annual income and assets are below the eligibility thresholds. These limits may change from year to year.

- Annual income is higher than the eligibility limit, but you support other family members in the same household; or if you live in Hawaii or Alaska.

	Individual	Couple
Income Limit	$19,320	$26,130
Resource Limit	$14,010	$27,950

Income and resource limits are for 2022

---

[19] We will repeat some of this information in Chapter 11.

Assets that count toward eligibility include:

- Cash and bank accounts including checking, savings, and certificates of deposit
- Real estate outside of your primary residence
- Stocks and bonds including U.S. Savings Bonds
- Mutual funds and IRAs

How to Apply:

- Online: *www.socialsecurity.gov/extrahelp*
- Call Social Security: 800-772-1213
- Apply at a local Social Security office

Social Security will forward your information to your state to ascertain Medicare Savings Plan eligibility. The state will contact you. After approval, if you do not select a Part D plan, Medicare will choose one for you.

WHAT'S NEXT?

After you have made your Part D choice and are in your enrollment period, you are ready to enroll in a plan:

- Contact a broker or agent who understands Part D plans
- Go to *Medicare.gov*, do your research, and make a choice
- Call a plan and enroll on the phone
- Go online and enroll in a plan

Obviously, as brokers, we enjoy hearing from new clients and will treat you with professionalism and use our knowledge to find the best match for your needs. Request a free consultation: *https://www.professormedicare.com/request-a-quote.*

OPINION

As U.S. drug prices vary wildly, with some branded medications priced painfully high, many individuals and some politicians are demanding more stringent controls on how pharmaceutical companies charge us. When Part D took effect in 2006, there was no provision for CMS to negotiate drug prices. Thirteen years later, CMS still has no ability to negotiate with drug manufacturers.

Our drug spending per capita is more than $1000 per year, yet the French and Germans pay half that even though we use fewer and cheaper drugs.[20] Think the pharmaceutical industry has anything to do with that?

In 2019 more than 1,300 Big Pharma lobbyists spent more than $155 million to pressure members of Congress to nod and wink in their direction. Does your senator or representative accept money from the lobby? Visit *www.opensecrets.org.* You may be surprised by what you find.

SUMMARY

Unbridled prescription drug prices are leaving inflation in the dust. But enrolling in a Part D plan can help Medicare beneficiaries control their drug spending. Understanding the plans, when to enroll, how drugs are tiered, rules for coverage, and how to get help with costs can make the process less

---

[20] Simon F. Haeder, "Why the US Has Higher Drug Prices than Other Countries," *The Conversation,* February 7, 2019, https://theconversation.com/why-the-us-has-higher-drug-prices-than-other-countries-111256.

daunting and ensure that you choose the right plan to ride through retirement.

CHAPTER QUESTIONS

1. When will you find out about yearly changes for your Part D plan?
2. Do all plans charge a deductible?
3. What costs more: A Tier 2 or Tier 4 medication?
4. Will there be a copay for a shingles vaccination?
5. Do all Medicare Advantage plans have a Part D?

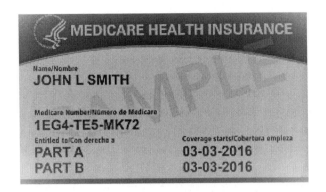

CHAPTER 8

ENROLLMENT

When should you enroll in Medicare? It's simple. You turn 65 and sign up . . . right?

It's complicated.

To be eligible for Medicare, you must be 65 and a legal resident of the United States for five years in a row. People under 65 with a qualifying disability are also eligible. If you have a diagnosis of end-stage renal disease or ALS, you qualify at any age.

So If you are 65, non-disabled, no longer working, and have lived in the United States for five consecutive years, yes, you sign up during your Initial Enrollment Period (IEP).

But if you currently receive Social Security or Railroad benefits or are disabled you will be automatically enrolled when you become eligible.

If you still work and have an employer health plan or didn't apply when you first became eligible, you will need to follow a few extra steps.

It is important to know Medicare's rules so you don't miss your windows of eligibility. Failing to sign up or letting some coverage lapse can result in permanent fines (see Appendix E).

If you don't sign up during your IEP or find you need to change your coverage, Medicare offers other enrollment periods throughout the year, each with its own stipulations about what you may add or change.

Regardless of your situation, *Professor Medicare* will help you sort through your Medicare options, get you signed up, and set you on a clear path forward.

INITIAL ENROLLMENT PERIOD (IEP/ICEP)[21]

One of the most important timelines in your Medicare experience is the Initial Enrollment Period. It applies only to the time when you first become eligible for Medicare.

You have seven months to complete Medicare enrollment. This includes three months before your birthday, the month you turn 65, and three months after. The best time to apply is three months before your 65th birthday. After the first four months, the start of coverage and coordinating an MA, SUPP, or Part D plan will be delayed.

---

[21] IEP refers to plans that include Part D. ICEP is for those that do not. For purposes of illustration, we will refer only to IEP.

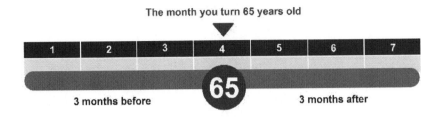

The month you turn 65 years old

| 1 | 2 | 3 | 4 | 5 | 6 | 7 |

65

3 months before   3 months after

For example, if your birthday is September 15, your IEP begins June 1 and ends December 31. If you sign up before your birthday month, your coverage will begin in September. However, if you delay signing up until November, your coverage will not start until February—three months after you signed up.

You enroll in A (if paid for) and/or B during this month	Start of Coverage
Month you turn 65	*1 month after sign up*
One month after turning 65	*2 months after sign up*
Two months after turning 65	*3 months after sign up*
Three months after turning 65	*3 months after sign up*
General Enrollment Jan 1–March 31	*July 1*

Exception: If you were born on the first day of the month, your Medicare will begin the prior month. For example, if you were born on August 1, you will have a July 1 Medicare start date.

HOW TO ENROLL

It takes 15–30 minutes to apply. You will need:

- Date and place of birth (plus Permanent Resident Card number if you are not a U.S. citizen)
- Social Security number
- Medicaid number, if applicable (plus start and end dates)
- Employment and health insurance start and end dates for the person currently covered by employer group health insurance

Where to enroll:

- Online at *www.ssa.gov/Medicare* or *www.Medicare.gov* (only if you were born in this country and are not receiving SS or Railroad benefits)
- Call Social Security at 800-772-1213
- Make an appointment and visit a Social Security office if allowed

In two to three weeks you will get a letter confirming your Medicare start date. Your card will follow soon. Once your enrollment is confirmed, you can choose an MA or SUPP plan to start on the 1st of your eligible month of coverage.

WHAT TO SIGN UP FOR

Parts A and B: When you apply for Medicare, you are enrolled in Parts A and B (Original Medicare). Part A has zero premium if you or your spouse paid into Medicare for at least 40 quarters.

But Part B charges a premium of $170.10 per month (more for higher incomes).[22] You may decline this coverage when you apply.

Or, if you have an employer plan that offers better benefits and/or cheaper costs, you may keep that and suspend Part B until you quit your job. To suspend Part B, follow the directions in your enrollment confirmation letter.

If you do not enroll in Part B during your IEP, you have another chance each year during the General Enrollment Period (GEP) from January 1–March 31. Coverage begins July 1 of the year you enroll. However, coverage lapses may thereafter incur a monthly penalty.

Part C: You may sign up for MA plans during your IEP or AEP, October 15–December 7.

Part D: You may sign up during your IEP or OEP. If coverage lapses for more than 63 days, you may thereafter incur a monthly penalty. If you have limited resources and income, you may be eligible for extra help with Part D expenses.

HOW AND WHEN CAN I CHANGE MY PLAN?

You may add or change coverage during Medicare's other enrollment periods (see below). Each has its own guidelines.

SPECIAL ENROLLMENT PERIODS (SEP)

You may qualify to change your coverage during a Special Enrollment Period if your life or plan changes significantly. These common situations might trigger an SEP:

---

[22] Premium, deductible, and fine numbers you see are for 2022.

- You move outside your plan's service area
- You move back to the U.S. after living in another country
- You move into or out of an institution such as a nursing home
- You were released from jail
- You lose your Medicaid coverage
- Your plan changes its contract with Medicare
- You qualify for a Low-Income Subsidy (LIS) to pay for prescription drugs
- You left an employer plan

Check the appendix or *www.medicare.gov* for more on Special Enrollment Periods.

GENERAL ENROLLMENT PERIOD (GEP)

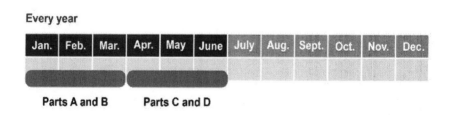

If you miss your IEP and aren't eligible for an SEP, you can still sign up for Part A and/or Part B between January 1–March 31 each year. Coverage will start July 1. Remember that you may pay a penalty for late enrollment.

What happens if you miss your IEP and don't have an employer plan or other creditable coverage?

Here is what one client encountered when she dealt with a delayed Part B enrollment:

CASE STUDY MARIE

We got a call from Marie, who had seen our *Professor Medicare* listing on Google. She was distressed. She was 69 years old and a fit and healthy person until she was hit with a diagnosis of lymphoma.

But she had no health coverage. Since her health was excellent at 65, she had decided there was no sense in paying premiums for a health care plan she would never use. She imagined she would never have a serious health issue. She called us in November after getting her new diagnosis.

Marie was also operating under a false assumption regarding enrollment. A friend had told her she could enroll in Medicare during AEP, but that was not true.

She could change plans during AEP if she had a plan in force, but for an initial Medicare enrollment, she would have to wait until January 1–March 31 to enroll. This is the GEP, and it's for those who missed IEP but had no employer or creditable coverage.

But even though Marie could enroll during the January to March window, her Medicare A and B would not start until July 1. She would have months without coverage, and she was dealing with a serious disease.

ANNUAL ENROLLMENT PERIOD (AEP)

Every year

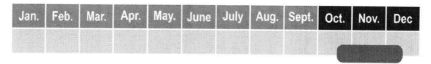

October 15 - December 7

The Annual Enrollment Period occurs every year from October 15–December 7. This is when you should compare your current coverage with your future healthcare needs and new plans that have become available. Coverage changes take effect the following January 1.

During AEP, you may:

- Change from Original Medicare, Part A and Part B, to an MA plan
- Change from an MA plan to Original Medicare, Part A and Part B
- Move from one MA plan to another
- Disenroll from an MA plan and enroll in a SUPP
- Disenroll from a SUPP and enroll in an MA plan
- Enroll in Part D
- Change your Part D plan

OPEN ENROLLMENT PERIOD (OEP)

Every year

Jan.	Feb.	Mar.	Apr.	May	June	July	Aug.	Sept.	Oct.	Nov.	Dec.

January 1 - March 31

If this wasn't complicated enough, in 2019 Medicare added the Open Enrollment Period from January 1–March 31. Because many people misunderstand MA plans, the government created this enrollment period as a safe "do over" if beneficiaries find they chose the wrong plan.

During OEP you may:

- Switch from one MA plan to another
- Disenroll from an MA plan and return to Original Medicare, with or without a Part D drug plan

Note that you cannot change from one Part D plan to another during OEP.

5-STAR ENROLLMENT

The Center for Medicare Services (CMS) rates MAs from 1–5 stars. To entice subscribers into these high-quality plans, Medicare permits them to drop an MA or SUPP anytime and enroll in a 5-star plan. These plans can be sold all year, but you can only make one change per year.

TIPS FROM PROFESSOR MEDICARE

There are two little-known but very useful ways to enroll in a SUPP outside of normal enrollment periods.

MA TO SUPP

Anyone who has turned 65 and enrolled in Part A can use what is called a one-time "trial right" to "try" a SUPP.

Medicare gives you one year and 63 days to disenroll from your MA plan and enroll in a SUPP with no health questions asked.

Why would you want to do this? Here is a real-life example from one of our clients. Beatrice turned 65 and enrolled in an MA plan. Three months later she called and said she would need at least two serious back surgeries with hospitalizations, then stays in skilled nursing facilities, with months of rehab to follow.

We moved her from the MA plan to a SUPP plus Part D plan and she saved a substantial amount of money. The next AEP, she was healthy and well and moved back to the MA plan.

SUPP TO MA TO SUPP

Similarly, if you enrolled in a SUPP plan and you changed to an MA plan during AEP, you have a year and 63 days to move back to that same SUPP plan if you are not happy with the MA plan. No questions asked.

Again, here is an actual example of how one of our clients used this right:

CASE STUDY GEETA

Geeta began with a SUPP, then moved to an MA plan during AEP.

About three months later she had a shoulder replacement, but with complications. She faced several more tests and lengthy rehab appointments at $40 each along with specialist appointments at $50 each. She could need another surgery.

Faced with all the copays and surgery charges, she wondered if she could do anything to lessen the financial burden.

Yes! We moved her back to her Plan F SUPP and a year later when she was healthy again, she returned to her MA plan during AEP.

You can use this option only once.

SUMMARY

One of the most common complaints we hear is that people are confused about when to sign up for Medicare. Some people fear a fine for not signing up when turning 65. But if you are employed at a company with more than 20 employees, there is no need to sign up at 65 if the plan meets IRS guidelines.

Others may think they can keep COBRA for a full 18 months and then sign up for Medicare. Wrong—although COBRA may last 18 months, you only have eight months after turning 65 to sign up for Part B.

Those are just a couple of examples of why it's advisable to consult with a professional regarding your Medicare enrollment.

We have covered a lot of ground in this enrollment chapter. The point is to give you enough information so you can feel comfortable with your decision about when to enroll in Medicare.

Remember in the Introduction, our first important question was "When Do I Enroll in Medicare?" This chapter should help you answer that question.

Some circumstances are complicated. We have seen more than a few. If that is your situation, give *Professor Medicare* a call or email with your questions. There is never a fee for our services.

CHAPTER QUESTIONS

1. How long is the Initial Enrollment Period?
2. Where do you go to enroll in Medicare when turning 65?
3. What is the Part B monthly premium?
4. Can you change plans during the year? When?
5. What is 5-Star Enrollment?

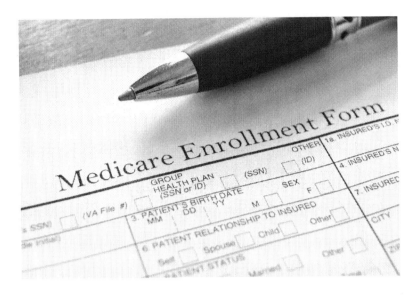

CHAPTER 9

ENROLLMENT CONDITIONS

For most people, Medicare enrollment is simple and takes only 15–30 minutes. But certain situations may affect how or when you sign up for Medicare. Some enroll you automatically with no application needed. For others, you will want to do a cost/benefit analysis to determine the best plan and then pay close attention to its deadlines.

If you already receive Social Security or Railroad benefits, are on disability, or plan to continue working after you turn 65, this chapter will walk you down the right path and help you make the best healthcare decisions for you and your family.

IF YOU ALREADY RECEIVE SOCIAL SECURITY OR RAILROAD BENEFITS

If you already receive Social Security or Railroad Retirement Board benefits, you don't need to apply for Medicare at all! You will be automatically enrolled in Medicare Parts A and B when you become eligible. Social Security will mail you a card. No further action is necessary unless you wish to decline or suspend Part B (see "If You Plan to Continue Working After 65" below).

IF YOU ARE ON DISABILITY

If you are under 65 and have been on disability for 24 months, your Medicare starts automatically on month 25 of your disability. No further action is required by you.

IF YOU HAVE RENAL DISEASE OR ALS

If you have end stage renal disease or ALS, enrollment is based on the timing of your diagnosis and possibly other factors.

IF YOU PLAN TO CONTINUE WORKING AFTER 65

Not everyone retires at 65. If you will continue to work, must you still sign up for Medicare? Can you keep your employer healthcare plan or should you switch to Medicare? The answers may depend on how large your company is and what the costs and benefits are.

If your employer has more than 20 full-time employees with a healthcare plan that meets IRS guidelines, then you do not have to enroll in Medicare upon turning 65. Always check with your benefits administrator to determine whether your employer plan meets IRS guidelines. If your current plan's costs and benefits make it preferable to Medicare, you can keep it (and suspend Plan B) until you retire or choose to drop it.

Once you do retire, you may apply for Medicare during a Special Enrollment Period (SEP) any time during the year.

If your company has fewer than 20 full-time employees, you must enroll in Medicare A and B. Medicare will become your primary coverage. If you don't enroll, you will be subject to a fine once you do sign up (see Appendix E).

IF YOU ARE LEAVING AN EMPLOYER PLAN

If you are retiring and leaving an employer plan, you'll need to begin the process before your actual retirement date. Certain forms must be filled out by your benefits administrator and then taken to Social Security.

Here is an example of a 68-year-old with an employer plan. She wants to retire and enroll in Medicare. Let's say she wants to retire on August 31 and start her Medicare A and B on September 1. Here is what she needs to do:

1. Start the process at least two months before retiring: e.g., in June for August 31 retirement.
2. Take *CMS Form L564* to the benefits administrator at work.
3. Once the *L564* is complete, take it and *Form 40B* to a Social Security office (you may have to make an appointment and that could take a month, or you may walk into the office and get immediate service). You can also call Security at 800-772-1213.
4. It takes two to three weeks to get a letter from Medicare stating your dates of coverage. Your

Medicare card follows the letter. Once you get that letter, you can enroll in an MA or SUPP plan and a standalone Part D plan.

You can find those forms and an explanation here: *https://www.professormedicare.com/medicare-eligible-employees.*

TIPS FOR ENROLLING AFTER LEAVING EMPLOYMENT

- When you have the administrator complete the *L564,* ask for the evidence of drug coverage too. Get it all done at once.

- When you turn 65, enroll in Part A if you have worked and contributed for 40 quarters. Why? First, it won't cost you anything, and second, it will not delay you enrolling in Part B when you leave your employer plan.

  We have had clients go to the Social Security office with all their correct paperwork for Part B and tried to enroll in Part A. They are sent away and told to sign up for A first and come back after Social Security approves Part A.

  To avoid that hassle, enroll in Part A when you turn 65. Your employer plan will continue to be primary if the company has more than 20 employees.

- Be aware of the timelines as discussed. Missing one can be costly. For example, if you miss enrolling in Part B during IEP or the eight months after leaving an employer plan, you must wait until the next GEP from Jan 1–March 31. And then your plan will not start until July 1.

IF YOU HAVE FAMILY MEMBERS ON YOUR EMPLOYEE PLAN

The choice of whether to keep an employer plan or enroll in Medicare may be made for you if you need healthcare coverage for family members. One of our clients, Dan, was about to turn 65 and planned to work a few more years. He called us to help determine if he should stay with his employer plan or move to Medicare.

Dan's wife, Sally, was 61 and their daughter, Bridget, was 20. On his employer plan the monthly premium for all three was approximately $600. Their deductible was $500 per person and $1500 for the family. It was a decent employer plan. They had no major health issues or costly medications.

If Dan moved to Medicare, his wife and child would have to find an ACA plan on the state health exchange. We found that there was a huge cost difference if they left his employer plan:

	Current Plan	Family Minus Dan	Medicare Advantage	Medigap
PREMIUM	$600	$1654	$0	$105
PART B PREMIUM			$170.10	$170.10
PART D PREMIUM			$0	$22.70
DEDUCTIBLE	$500	$2000	$0	$233
% AFTER DEDUCTIBLE	10%	20%	NA	0
MAXOOP	$3000	$6700	$4400	NA
Monthly Total	$600	$1654	$170.10	$297.80
Yearly Total	$7200	$19,848	$2041.20	$3806.60

If Dan kept his employer plan and postponed enrolling in Part B, he would continue to pay $600 a month.

If Dan enrolled in Part B and an MA plan and then enrolled Sally and Bridget in a plan on the ACA Exchange, their combined monthly premiums would jump to $1824.10.

In addition, the ACA plan benefits were not as rich as those in the employer plan. Simply stated, Medicare plus ACA provided less coverage for an additional $1224.10 a month in premiums. It was an easy decision for Dan and Sally. They kept the employer plan and Dan will enroll in Part B when he quits working.

Our cost chart above shows only the premium, deductible, and max out-of-pocket differences. For Dan and Sally, we prepared a detailed analysis of yearly healthcare and drug costs. We suggest you do this too. No one knows what their future healthcare or drug costs may be, but we can start with today's real numbers. Look at your health expenses last year and use that as a guideline.

If Dan enrolls in Medicare after his IEP, below are the timelines he needs to use. The first shows his SEP opening. The second is for enrolling in an MA and Part D.

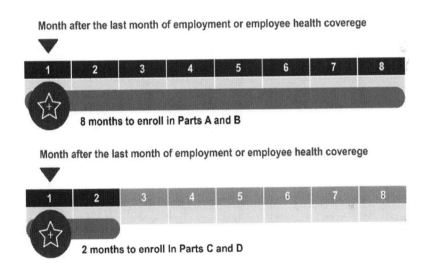

Month after the last month of employment or employee health coverege

8 months to enroll in Parts A and B

Month after the last month of employment or employee health coverege

2 months to enroll In Parts C and D

SEPs for Enrollment in Original Medicare, MAs, and Part D When Moving from an Employer Plan

IF YOU NEED PART D DRUG COVERAGE AFTER AN EMPLOYER PLAN

If you start your Medicare Part D after IEP when you leave an employer plan, you need to prove you had creditable drug coverage. Once you have enrolled in a standalone Part D plan or one associated with an MA plan, the plan will send you a letter asking for evidence of coverage. You will then ask your employer's benefits administrator to provide, on company letterhead, the dates of your coverage from age 65 under the employer plan.

If you do not enroll in Part D during IEP, you may be subject to a permanent monthly fine (see appendix E).

IF YOU ARE ELIGIBLE FOR COBRA AFTER AN EMPLOYER PLAN

Once you retire, COBRA coverage may be available for you. It continues your employer plan insurance for up to 18 months. However, in most cases, COBRA is more expensive than Medicare. If you have family members who are under 65, a careful cost analysis and comparison of coverage is necessary so you can make an intelligent decision. There is a limit to how long you can have COBRA without incurring a fine.

Don't wait until your 18 months of COBRA ends to enroll in Part B. Start the Medicare enrollment process about two months before ending your employment. Once you become eligible for Medicare at 65, you have eight months to sign up for Part B without a penalty.

To sign up for Part B while you're employed or during the eight months after employment ends, complete an *Application for Enrollment in Part B (CMS-40B)* and a *Request for Employment Information (CMS-L564)*.

If You Need a SUPP After an Employee Plan

What about enrolling in a SUPP? Open enrollment for SUPPs lasts six months. It starts with the month Part B becomes active and runs for five more months.

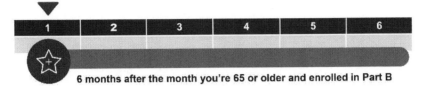

65 or older and enrolled in Part B

| 1 | 2 | 3 | 4 | 5 | 6 |

6 months after the month you're 65 or older and enrolled in Part B

SUMMARY

Some circumstances require you to follow specific timelines or procedures that differ from standard Medicare enrollment. If you already receive Social Security or Railroad benefits or are on disability, you will be automatically enrolled with no action necessary on your part. If you continue to work, you'll need to decide whether to keep your employer healthcare plan or switch to Medicare. Particularly if your plan covers other family members, this may require a comprehensive comparison of the benefits and costs of each option.

Knowing Medicare's guidelines and your options will ensure that you sign up for the appropriate benefits in a timely manner. Some situations are complicated, and you may want to seek professional advice. *Professor Medicare* is always glad to help, and there is never a fee for our services.

CHAPTER QUESTIONS

1. If you already receive Social Security, do you have to sign up for Medicare?
2. If you plan to keep working after 65, can you keep your employer health plan?
3. When you leave an employer health plan and begin Medicare, what two forms do you need to file?
4. What is the timeline for enrolling in Medicare when leaving an employer plan?
5. How do you prove your employer drug coverage was "creditable"?

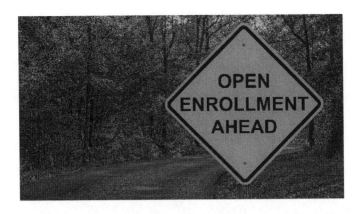

CHAPTER 10

CHANGING PLANS

When you marry, you commit "'til death us do part." But just because you sign up for a certain Medicare Advantage plan, Supplement, or Part D plan during your Initial Enrollment Period, it doesn't mean you're stuck with it for life. When your situation changes, you can switch to a new plan that better meets your needs.

For example, if you have an MA plan and move out of the plan's coverage area, you will need to change plans. If a new plan offers more or better benefits than your plan, that's a reason to switch. If you are pinched financially and don't want to pay SUPP and Part D premiums, that is also motivation to move. If your plan closes, you will have to select a new one. If your Part D plan doesn't give you the best pricing on your meds, that's grounds for a change.

Since we are dealing with Medicare rules, it is not simply a matter of ordering a new policy online. Guidelines and timelines dictate when you may switch plans and the steps you must follow. MA plans, SUPPs, and Part D plans all have different rules for moving. But a little effort will ensure you continue to have the best coverage. And we can help.

First let's look at SUPPs.

CHANGING SUPPLEMENT COMPANIES OR PLANS

SUPPs have an OEP, which is the month your Part B starts plus five additional months. After that you can change your SUPP at any time during the year. However, you may have to deal with health-related questions and can be denied coverage. We don't see a lot of movement with our SUPP clients. All plans have yearly age-related premium increases, but they are generally modest. An increase of 10%–20% might motivate an exodus, but that kind of increase is rare.

GUARANTEED ISSUE

If you want to change plans and have a Guaranteed Issue circumstance, you are exempt from answering medical questions and guaranteed acceptance in the new plan. We have posted the Guaranteed Issue explanations in Chapter 5.

MOVE FROM SUPP TO MA PLAN

If you want to change from a SUPP to an MA plan, you can do so during AEP from October 15–December 7.

MOVE BACK TO SUPP FROM MA PLAN

What if you leave a SUPP to join an MA plan and want to move back to your SUPP? You have one year after beginning your new MA plan to return to the same SUPP with the same company you had before. Medicare wants to make sure you are happy with your MA plan.

CHANGING MEDICARE ADVANTAGE (MA) PLANS

Every fall, Medicare Advantage plans ramp up their marketing efforts. You will receive mailers and see/hear advertisements on various media and the internet. MA plans cover nearly 35% of all Medicare beneficiaries and that market share expands yearly. New MA plans are created every year and one entering your area may have more robust benefits than your current plan. It is a competitive marketplace for MA plans.

CHANGING YOUR MA DURING THE ANNUAL ENROLLMENT PERIOD (AEP)

October 15–December 7 is the Annual Enrollment Period, with all plans starting on January 1. You can change your mind as many times as you wish during this time, but your last choice is the one that begins on January 1. Here are the changes you can make during AEP:

- Move from one MA to another
- Move from an MA plan with no Part D coverage to one with Part D
- Move from an MA with Part D to a plan without drug coverage
- Move from an MA plan to Original Medicare

- Move from an MA plan to Original Medicare and then a SUPP
- Move from Original Medicare to an MA plan

In our Metro Denver, Colorado, market, there are 8 MA carriers available for 2022. Each carrier has multiple plans. There are HMOs, PPOs, DSNP, CSNP, and ISNP, to name a few. Makes my head spin.

Before October 1 agents are only permitted to speak in generalities about what is coming for AEP. After October 1 we can talk about specific plans and benefits but must wait until the 15th to enroll clients. It is a mass of information, but our job is to make it clear and easy for our valued clients and new clients to understand.

If you are in another state, monitor the marketplace. Call your agent and ask about good coverage options going forward.

Until 2019 AEP was the most popular time to move from or to MA plans. Medicare added OEP in 2019.

CHANGING YOUR MA DURING THE OPEN ENROLLMENT PERIOD (OEP)

The Open Enrollment Period replaced the Medicare Advantage Disenrollment Period which ran from January 1–February 14. It allowed beneficiaries to disenroll from an MA plan and move to Original Medicare. Medicare eliminated the Disenrollment Period in favor of the more expansive OEP. Here is what you can do during OEP from January 1–March 31:

- Change MA plans
- Leave your MA plan and go to Original Medicare

- Apply for a SUPP and a stand-alone Part D plan

This means you have from October 15–March 31 to change MA plans or go back to Original Medicare.

CHANGING A PART D PLAN

Outside of your IEP or a SEP, the only time you can change Part D plans is during the yearly AEP. An SEP expands your enrollment ability. However, if an MA plan or Part D plan has a 5-star rating, you can move to it any time during the year—but only once a year.

SPECIAL ENROLLMENT PERIOD (SEP) FOR MA AND PART D

Here are some situations when you can use a Special Enrollment Period to enroll in MA plans and Part D plans:

- You qualify for extra help
- You move out of your plan's area
- Your plan is no longer contracted with Medicare
- You move into or out of an institution
- You lose creditable drug coverage or your plan is not creditable

SUMMARY

It is possible to move from one MA, SUPP, or Part D plan to another, but moving is not as easy as it sounds. Certain moves must be made during specific enrollment periods. Others may require health qualification.

If you want to change your plan, make sure your providers accept the new plan. Check your drug costs too. At first glance, a new plan may look great, but if you drill down, you may find some meds are more costly or not even covered. The network may be much smaller than what you are using and that means fewer choices.

We have provided the basics of plan changes. Before making any move, be sure to research the full details. A knowledgeable agent such as *Professor Medicare* can help you with this.

CHAPTER QUESTIONS

1. Can you change your Supplement Plan G to a Plan N whenever you want?

2. Can you change your Part D when you switch Supplements?

3. If you just qualified for a Low-Income Subsidy, can you change Medicare Advantage plans?

4. My neighbor told me I can change my drug plan during the Open Enrollment Period from January 1– March 31. Is this true?

5. Can I change from a Supplement to a Medicare Advantage plan during the Annual Enrollment Period in the fall?

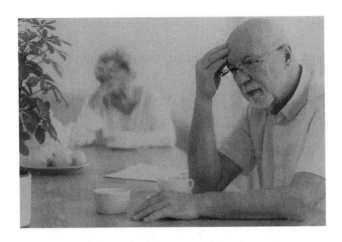

CHAPTER 11

EXTRA HELP

Money makes up only one-third of our *Big Three* of *Money-Health-Relationships,* but it seems to have an outsized influence, especially for seniors living on fixed incomes.

Seniors and retirees look at life differently than folks who are still working and only planning for retirement. For most of us, the reality of retirement is a far cry from what we imagined at age 40 or 50.

The Transamerica Center for Retirement Studies commissioned a survey of seniors' attitudes toward retirement. Its report, *A Precarious Existence: How Today's Retirees Are Financially Faring in Retirement,* was published in December 2018 and is available online. Some findings were sobering:

- Only 46% of retirees agree they have a large enough nest egg while 30% strongly disagree.

- One in three say their financial situation has declined since entering retirement. 42% say it has stayed the same.

- 59% say they spend less in retirement.

- 66% say Social Security will be their primary source of income.

- Retirees report an annual household income of $32,000 (estimated median). 25% have a household income less than $25,000. 15% have an income of $100,000 or more.

- Many are still paying off household debt such as car loans, credit cards, student loans, and medical debt. 28% have mortgage debt.

- 46% of retirees do not have a retirement strategy.

What if you need assisted living or long-term care? These costs are sky high and inflating yearly. In the Denver Metro Area, the average monthly costs are:

Home Health Care Aide	$5243
Assisted Living	$4700
Nursing Home Semi-Private Room	$8365
Nursing Home Private Room	$9520

Scary stuff, eh? Only a minority of retirees have the financial resources to deal with a major health decline. What happens if your income drops or you run out of savings? What if you began Medicare but have limited resources to pay the costs? We will show you how and where to get some help.

Two main government-sponsored programs help enrollees pay for premiums and out-of-pocket costs based on income: Low-Income Subsidy (LIS) for Part D and Medicare Savings Programs (MSP) for Parts A and B.

LOW-INCOME SUBSIDY (LIS)

The Low-Income Subsidy is a government program that helps people with low incomes pay Part D monthly premiums, annual deductibles, coinsurance, and copayments.

Dependent upon a beneficiary's income and resources, the subsidy averages $4900 per year. Being in the program eliminates the Part D Donut Hole or Coverage Gap and late enrollment fines.

ELIGIBILITY

You may qualify for the LIS available under Medicare Part D if your:

- Annual income and assets are below the eligibility thresholds. These limits may change from year to year.
- Annual income is higher than the eligibility limit, but you support other family members in the same household; or if you live in Alaska or Hawaii.

	Individual	Couple
Income Limit	$19,320	$26,130
Resource Limit	$14,010	$27,950

Income and resource limits are from 2022.

Assets that count toward eligibility include:

- Cash and bank accounts including checking, savings, and certificates of deposit
- Real estate outside of your primary residence
- Stocks and bonds including U.S. Savings Bonds
- Mutual funds and IRAs

How to apply:

- Online: *www.socialsecurity.gov/extrahelp*
- Call Social Security: 800-772-1213
- Apply at a local Social Security office

Social Security will forward your information to your state to ascertain LIS eligibility. The state will contact you. After approval, if you do not select a Part D plan, Medicare will choose one for you.

MEDICARE SAVINGS PROGRAMS (MSP)

Four different Medicare Savings Programs—QMB, SLMB, QI-1, and QDWI—help beneficiaries with limited income pay Part A and/or Part B premiums and out-of-pocket costs. Each has specific requirements and income limits. If you have employment income, you may still qualify for benefits even if your income is higher than listed limits.

Here is the qualification chart from 2021:

	Individual income limit	Married couple income limit	Individual resource limit	Couple resource limit
QMB	$1,094	$1,472	$9,470	$14,960
SLMB	$1,308	$1,762	$9,470	$14,960
QI	$1,469	$1,980	$9,470	$14,960
QDWI	$2,167	$2,924	$4,000	$6,000

BENEFITS

Each MSP offers a specific package to cover premiums, deductibles, copays, and coinsurance.

QMB: Part A and Part B premiums, copays, and coinsurance

SLMB: Part B premium

QI: Part B premium

QDWI: Part A premium

RESOURCE LIMITS

To qualify for an MSP, you must meet certain income requirements. Countable Resources include:

- Money in a checking or savings account
- Stocks and bonds
- Money in an IRA, annuity, or trust

Countable Resources do *not* include:

- Your home
- One car
- Burial plot
- Up to $1500 set aside for burial expenses
- Furniture
- Other personal and household items

HOW TO APPLY FOR ASSISTANCE

If you live in Colorado and think you qualify for assistance, apply to your county Department of Human Services: *www.Colorado.gov/cdhs/contact-your-county*.

If you live in another state, go to your county Senior Services or Health and Human Services. Every state has a Senior Health Insurance Assistance Program (SHIP) office. You can find a wealth of resources at SHIP. Medicare provides a search engine to help you locate your state resources: *https://www.medicare.gov/Contacts/*.

You can also apply for LIS or MSP online at *https://secure.ssa.gov/i1020/start* or by calling Social Security at 800-772-1213.

SUMMARY

We all envision a retirement of good health and leisure—pursuing hobbies, traveling, volunteering, spending time with family and friends. However, a sudden decline in health or financial resources can undo even the best planning and decimate your savings.

Medicare helps countless seniors receive the healthcare they need at a reasonable cost. But if your financial situation makes it hard to pay your premiums, deductibles, copays, and coinsurance, additional help is available.

The Low-Income Subsidy Program covers some of your Part D expenses. A variety of Medicare Savings Programs cover different combinations of Part A and B costs.

It's good to have a safety net as we age. Both LIS and MSP give us good options if our resources shrink.

CHAPTER QUESTIONS

1. True or False: 75% of retirees have a retirement strategy.
2. Can anyone qualify for a Low-Income Subsidy?
3. Will the QMB level of a Medicare Savings Program pay for the Part B premium?
4. Does an auto or home count as a resource when applying for extra help?
5. Where should you apply for a Medicare Savings Program?

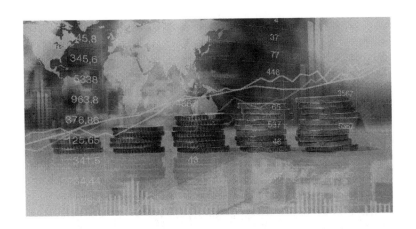

CHAPTER 12

CHARGES FOR HIGHER INCOMES

No one likes to pay extra. But Medicare's IRMAA is one surcharge every senior would love to qualify for.

If your income is above $91,000 ($182,000 for couples), Medicare requires you to pay more for monthly Part B and Part D premiums. Between 6%–7% of all beneficiaries are assessed an Income-Related Monthly Adjustment Amount (IRMAA).

Social Security determines how much more you will pay based on your tax returns. The IRS allows Social Security a two-year look-back at your most recent returns. For 2022, they look at your filing for tax year 2020. If you turn 65 or start your Part B in 2022, Social Security looks at your 2020 tax return.

Your Modified Adjusted Gross Income (MAGI) is the magic number. MAGI is your total Adjusted Gross Income (AGI) plus tax-exempt interest income. There is one amount for single filers and another for married couples filing jointly.

When we meet with new clients, we show the charts you will see below. Even though only a few enrollees will have IRMAA charges, it's good practice to mention it. No one wants to get a letter from the government telling them there is more to pay, right?

INCOME-RELATED MONTHLY ADJUSTMENT AMOUNT (IRMAA)

If you have to pay more, at least it should be easy to figure out, right? Yes! Determining your Income-Related Monthly Adjustment Amount is one of the easiest Medicare-related tasks.

The first chart you see is for Part B charges, the larger assessments. Although based on the same income numbers, Part D excess charges are much smaller. Wherever you fall in the IRMAA ranges, be prepared to deal with both amounts.

Here is the Part B IRMAA chart:

If your yearly income in 2020 (for what you pay in 2022) was			
File individual tax return	File joint tax return	File married & separate tax	You pay each month (in 2020)
$91,000 or less	$182,000 or less	$91,000 or less	$170.10
above $91,000 up to $114,000	above $182,000 up to $228,000	Not applicable	$238.10
above $114,000 up to $142,000	above $228,000 up to $284,000	Not applicable	$340.20
above $142,00 up to $170,000	above $284,000 up to $340,000	Not applicable	$442.30
$170,000 and less than $500,000	above $340,000 and less than $750,000	above $91,000 and less than $409,000	$544.30
$500,000 or above	$750,000 and above	$409,000 and above	$578.30

And IRMAA for Part D:

If your yearly income in 2020 (for what you pay in 2022) was			
File individual tax return	File joint tax return	File married & separate tax	You Pay each month (in 2020)
$91,000 or less	$182,000 or less	$91,000 or less	Your plan premium
above $91,000 up to $114,000	above $182,000 up to $228,000	Not applicable	$12.40 + your plan premium
above $114,000 up to $142,000	above $228,000 up to $284,000	Not applicable	$32.10 + your plan premium
above $142,000 up to $170,000	above $284,000 up to $340,000	Not applicable	$51.70 + your plan premium
$170,000 and less than $500,000	above $340,000 and less than $750,000	above $91,000 and less than $409,000	$71.30 + your plan premium
$500,000 or above	$750,000 and above	$409,000 and above	$77.90 + your plan premium

WHAT IF MY INCOME CHANGES?

Your income probably remains stable from year to year. However, investment income or sale of a property can suddenly bump you into a higher bracket. Will you have to pay the surcharge forever after?

No. Social Security calculates IRMAA every year. If your MAGI triggers a surcharge in 2020 but your income goes down in 2021, you will be automatically moved back to the lower category for 2023.

REQUEST FOR RECONSIDERATION

If a life-changing event causes your income to go down mid-year, and it makes a difference in the MAGI Social Security uses to calculate your premium charges, you can request a reconsideration. Here are situations that can warrant that:

- Marriage, divorce, or death of a spouse
- Either you or your spouse stopped working or cut down your work hours
- You or your spouse lost an income-producing property because of disaster or events beyond your control
- You or your spouse had a scheduled cessation, reorganization, or termination of an employee pension plan
- You or your spouse received a settlement from an employer or former employer because of their closing, bankruptcy, or reorganization

If any of the above apply to you, you need to provide documentation relating to the event.

To request reconsideration because of a life-changing event, use *Form SSA-44 Medicare Income-Related Monthly Adjustment Amount-Life-Changing Event,* available at *https://www.ssa.gov/forms/ssa-44-ext.pdf.* To get any SSA form, enter the form title in your search engine or go to *SSA.gov* and find the form.

After you complete the Life-Changing Event form, you can go to your local Social Security office or call 800-772-1123, TTY 800-325-0778, and ask for help.

APPEALS

What if you submitted your Life-Changing Event form but are not satisfied with the ruling from Social Security? You can appeal the decision online or in writing.

- For online appeals, go to *www.socialsecurity.gov/disability/appeal* and choose *"Request Non-Medical Consideration."*

- To make a written request, complete a *Request for Reconsideration—Form SSA-561-U2.* You can either call 800-772-1213, TTY 800-325-0778, or go to your local office with your appeal.

Be ready to provide lots of documentation to back up your claim to an appeal.

SUMMARY

An Income-Related Monthly Adjustment Amount is charged to Medicare beneficiaries with incomes over $91,000 individuals/$182,000 for couples. This is a surcharge added to the monthly premium for Parts B and D. Based upon your Modified Adjusted Gross Income, it fluctuates yearly as your income changes. If a life-changing event causes your income to drop, you can request that your IRMAA be reconsidered, and you may appeal the decision if not satisfied.

CHAPTER QUESTIONS

1. If I am applying for Medicare in 2022, will they look at my 2019 tax return?
2. My household income is $150,000. Will I have an IRMAA charge?
3. Is my income my AGI?
4. How much would my IRMAA be for Part B and Part D if our joint income is $300,000?
5. Can I appeal an IRMAA charge online?

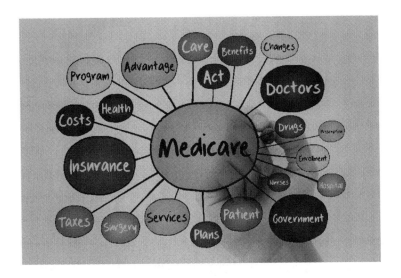

CHAPTER 13

SPECIAL TOPICS

To cover everything in the world of Medicare, this book would run thousands of pages. Our point was not to cover every nuance and special situation, but to explain the most important, most necessary topics concisely and accurately, using everyday language and offering real-world examples. A few topics didn't fit nicely into our other chapters, so we have collected them here.

CREATE ACCOUNTS

Some people panic when they need to locate some detail of their healthcare coverage, claims, or costs. They rifle through papers and files and rummage through drawers looking for that one particular document. But there's a way to instantly access all your information: set up a personal account online for each of your plans. You should create accounts for each of these programs:

- *www.mymedicare.gov*
- *www.ssa.gov*
- Your Medicare Advantage plan
- Your standalone Part D plan
- Your Medicare Supplement

Having these accounts at your fingertips will save you countless unnecessary phone calls or emails.

HOSPITAL OBSERVATION OR ADMISSION?

The gray area between an emergency room visit and an inpatient hospital admission causes a great deal of anxiety and anger.

For example, let's say you fall in the gym and slam into a hardwood floor. The fall knocks you dizzy, and you stumble. A friend takes you to the ER. The staff runs protocols and tests and finds you have a concussion. They are not sure if you have a brain bleed, so they order more tests. To be safe, they keep you overnight.

They place you in a hospital room, but you are not formally admitted. You are "under observation." Being under observation feels and appears exactly like being admitted. You are in a bed in the hospital, but you are not an inpatient—you are an outpatient.

Here is where it gets tricky. Medicare Part A covers you if you are an inpatient, but if you are not admitted, you will be under Part B. If you have an MA plan, you will have to pay outpatient coinsurance for the tests, medications, and literally everything that is part of your treatment.

Why is this? Hospitals are wary of admitting a patient and later have Medicare dispute that the admission was necessary. When that happens, hospitals must pay back their Part A charges.

Hospitals also want to avoid readmission penalties. In the past few years Medicare has cut payments when hospitals readmit patients within 30 days. To avoid that penalty, hospitals put patients in observation. If they go home the next day and come back later, it doesn't count as a readmission.

Even though patients get the same care under observation that they might get as inpatients, they will pay more (sometimes a lot more) for it. In 2016, Medicare spent over $3 billion for observation treatment. Clients paid their share.

WHAT CAN YOU DO?

When you are in hospital, ask whether they plan to admit you as an inpatient or under observation. Hospitals are now required to give patients the Medicare Outpatient Observation Notice within 36 hours if the patient is receiving observation services as an outpatient for 24 hours. Hospitals must explain this designation and its financial consequences face to face with the patient or patient's representative.

HOME HEALTHCARE

Homebound means it's hard for you to leave home, and if you do leave, you must have help. If you are homebound and require treatment for an injury or illness, Medicare covers a wide variety of services, both health and social, including:

- Therapy
- Skilled nursing care

- Care from a home health aide

Either Part A or B will cover your care for skilled nursing services and speech, occupational, and physical therapy. Skilled care is care performed or directly supervised by a professional.

BEGINNING HOME CARE

After examining you, your doctor will approve a plan of home care. He or she will sign a home health certification confirming that you are/will be homebound and need intermittent skilled care.

Every 60 days, your doctor must review and recertify your plan. You must receive care from a Medicare-certified Home Health Agency.

If you require skilled in-home nursing care, Medicare will also pay for an aide to help with personal care such as dressing, toileting, and eating. Note that you must be receiving skilled nursing care to have an aide for personal care.

Your doctor is the one who must write the order for your home care and once it is approved, Medicare will cover the care. This is true for MA clients as well as Original Medicare subscribers.

PROGRAM OF ALL-INCLUSIVE CARE FOR THE ELDERLY (PACE)

Medicare's Program of All-Inclusive Care for the Elderly (PACE) is for people over 55 who are frail and require nursing home-level care. PACE's philosophy is that whenever possible, people should be cared for in their homes or communities instead of in a nursing facility.

PACE is active in 31 states with more than 49,000 participants, 95% of whom live at home. Around 90% are eligible for both Medicare and Medicaid, or dual eligible. Averaging 76 years old, participants have multiple medical conditions, cognitive impairments, or significant or long-term health care needs.

When a participant enrolls, PACE creates an Interdisciplinary Team (IDT) including doctors, nurses, social workers, therapists, dieticians, personal care aides, drivers, and others. The IDT develops a care plan to respond 24/7 to the patient's needs.

Here are some services provided by PACE:

- Adult day care
- Lab and x-ray services
- Meals
- Dentistry
- Nursing home care
- Occupational or physical therapy
- Prescription drugs
- Emergency services

In Colorado, Health First Colorado operates the PACE program. You can contact your county senior services or health and human services department to get help with application and enrollment into PACE.

PREVENTIVE CARE

Preventive services help identify problems when they are small and potential problems before they impact your health. Medicare Part B covers these services, nearly always without any cost to patients. Here is a comprehensive list of Medicare preventive care services:

- One time "Welcome to Medicare" preventive visit—within the first 12 months you have Medicare Part B
- Yearly Wellness Visit—get this visit 12 months after your "Welcome to Medicare" preventive visit or 12 months after your Part B effective date
- Abdominal aortic aneurysm screening
- Alcohol misuse screening and counseling
- Bone mass measurement (bone density test)
- Cardiovascular disease (behavioral therapy)
- Cardiovascular screenings (cholesterol, lipids, triglycerides)
- Colorectal cancer screenings
- Depression screening
- Diabetes screening
- Diabetes self-management training
- Flu shot
- Glaucoma test
- Hepatitis B screening
- Hepatitis C screening
- HIV screening
- Lung cancer screening
- Mammogram (screening for breast cancer)
- Medical nutrition therapy services
- Medicare diabetes prevention program
- Obesity screening and counseling

- Pap test and pelvic exam (includes a breast exam)
- Pneumococcal shots
- Prostate cancer screening
- Sexually-transmitted infection screening and counseling
- Counseling to prevent tobacco use and tobacco-caused disease

For further details, access the CMS publication: *https://www.medicare.gov/Pubs/pdf/10110-Medicare-Preventive-Services.pdf?.*

SUMMARY

So . . . you have compared and chosen your Medicare parts and plans and enrolled in coverage. You're finished, right?

Maybe. Medicare is a comprehensive healthcare program and offers many options you might need but not be aware of, such as home and community healthcare and routine preventive care.

We have also shown you how to set up individual program accounts and what to do if a hospital proposes admitting you for observation. These extras will save you time and money and help you get the most from your Medicare enrollment.

CHAPTER QUESTIONS

1. Where can you access your claims history online?
2. Is PACE for anyone on Medicare?
3. Is there a charge for flu shots?

4. If you have a back operation and can't move enough to go to therapy sessions, what Medicare program can you use?

5. What part of Medicare covers you during a hospital "observation" stay?

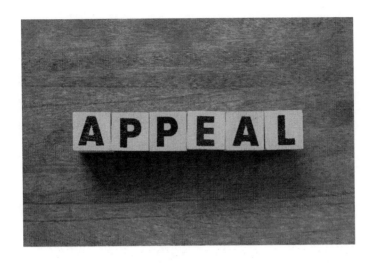

CHAPTER 14

APPEALS AND GRIEVANCES

Even a well-oiled machine breaks down occasionally.

Medicare is an enormous system, accounting for 15% of federal spending and covering about half of the healthcare expenses for more than 60 million Americans.[23] Its administrators work hard to ensure that the program runs smoothly and provides fair and equitable coverage.

The Centers for Medicare and Medicaid Services (CMS) standardize the plans that help consumers pay much of that other half through Medicare Advantage plans, Supplements, and Part D drug coverage. Its employees work hard to ensure that a

---

[23] "An Overview of Medicare," The Henry J. Kaiser Family Foundation, February 13, 2019, https://www.kff.org/medicare/issue-brief/an-overview-of-medicare/.

reasonable number and variety of plans comparable across states are available to consumers.

Private insurance companies underwrite the plans and make them available for sale. Their agents work hard to explain and compare plans to clients and match them with the combination of plans that best suits their needs and situations.

Despite the best efforts of so many committed people, sometimes things go wrong and your Medicare doesn't work the way you expect. You might encounter a clerical or coding error, a coverage disagreement, an operational glitch, or a plan misrepresentation.

Fortunately, Medicare addresses problems through Appeals and Grievances. Each addresses specific Medicare components through defined procedures. If you disagree with a payment or coverage decision made by Medicare, your health plan, or your Part D plan, you can file an Appeal. If you are not satisfied with the operations, activities, or behavior of a Medicare health plan, you may file a Grievance.

Before filing an appeal or grievance, it is a good idea to phone the provider, facility, or health plan to see if there was a clerical error. For example, if they charged you $200 for an office visit but your MA plan calls for only a $40 copay, you may learn that the visit was incorrectly coded. Coding errors cause the bulk of mistakes we see with billing. A simple phone call can easily and quickly resolve many issues and ease your anxiety.

APPEALS

Appeals are for disagreements over *payment and coverage decisions*. If you can't resolve your issue with phone calls, emails, or meetings, you may file an appeal. There are five levels of appeals. If you have an MA plan, your appeal will follow these steps:

Level 1: Contact your plan (your provider's office may help with this) and make a "request for consideration." Your MA plan informs you in writing how to file this request You will get a response in 30 days if it involves a request for service. If it's about a payment, the decision could take up to 60 days. Your doctor can request "expedited consideration" if waiting 30 days would jeopardize your health or life. If you are an inpatient, you can request an "immediate review" by a Quality Improvement Organization. If your plan does not decide in your favor or does not respond before the deadline, it automatically forwards your appeal to a Level 2 independent outside entity.

Level 2: The process here is different based on whether you are appealing Original Medicare A or B*, MA Part C, or Part D. So what is the process for each? If you disagree with the Level 2 decision, a "reconsidered determination," you can request that the Office of Medicare Hearings and Appeals (OMHA) review the decision.

Level 3: OMHA reviews your appeal. The independent adjudicator may decide your case without a hearing, or you may be granted a hearing before an administrative law judge. If you get a negative ruling at Level 3, you can take another step.

Level 4: The Medicare Appeals Council (MAC) is part of Health and Human Services and is independent of OMHA. You don't have an automatic right to a MAC review, but you can request one in writing or send it electronically. If you disagree with the council's decision and the monetary amount is at least $1560 (or $2000 in some areas), you can file a civil action at your local

Federal District Court. You must do this within 60 days of the Level 4 ruling.

* If you have a problem with Original Medicare, the Appeal process is different. Every three months you get a Medicare Summary Notice (MSN). If you don't agree with the numbers:

1. Circle the items you question. Be sure to write your reason for appealing on the notice or attach a sheet of paper.

2. Get the *Redetermination Request Form* from *cms.gov* or call Medicare at 800-633-4227. Make a copy. Send one copy to the contractor's address on the MSN. Be sure to file your Appeal within 120 days of the date you received your MSN.

3. If your first Appeal is denied, you can lodge another Appeal with a Qualified Independent Contractor. You can download the *Reconsideration Request Form* for this second level appeal at *cms.gov.* You must file this Appeal within 180 days of getting the denial of your first appeal.

4. If your Appeal fails with the Independent Contractor, you can proceed to Level 4. And if that fails, you have Level 5.

GRIEVANCES

Grievances are complaints about your *treatment.* Here are a few areas in which you would address a problem through a grievance:

- A doctor, hospital, or provider
- Your health or drug plan

- Quality of your care

- Your dialysis or kidney transplant care

- Durable medical equipment

To lodge a Grievance, contact the Beneficiary and Family Centered Care Quality Improvement Organization (BFCC-QIO) online at *www.keproqio.com*. In Colorado the number is 888-317-0891. You can also contact SHIP in Colorado at 888-696-7213 for Medicare questions and 800-503-5190 for errors or suspected fraud.

Outside Colorado, call your local SHIP office for help. You can find the number for your state at *https://www.medicare.gov/contacts/*.

Most people use their Medicare services for many years without any problems. We hope all goes smoothly for you too, but if problems occur, you have options to make things right.

You can file an appeal over payment or coverage decisions. If your dispute is over your care or treatment, you file a grievance. Make sure you follow the steps for either process.

As always, *Professor Medicare* can guide you through the dispute process.

CHAPTER QUESTIONS

1. If I think I was overcharged $100 for an office visit, should I file an appeal or a grievance?

2. The receptionist at my dermatologist's said she was tired of dealing with old people and their brown spots. Can I file a grievance?

3. If I am in hospital and was turned down for an operation, can my doctor get a fast appeal?

4. If there was a coding error on my bill, should I immediately file an appeal?

5. The company that delivers my oxygen is never on time, and I often have to call several times to get it. Is this grounds for an appeal or a grievance?

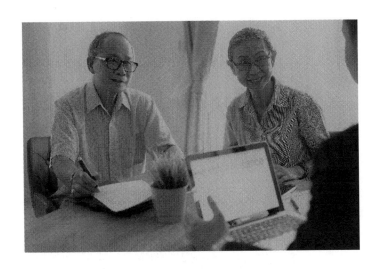

CHAPTER 15

WORKING WITH AN AGENT

It seems everyone is into DIY these days. You can find instructions online or in a book for anything from fixing a leaky faucet to building a bookcase to managing your anxiety.

We wrote this book for do-it-yourselfers who want to go at their own pace to educate themselves about Medicare options. After reading it you should be able to make an informed decision about coverage. However, because each part and plan has so many rules and conditions, it can be helpful to consult with an agent, if only to confirm that you have selected the right combination. Experienced agents like *Professor Medicare* know just what to ask to guide you through your plan assessment.

There is no charge for this service.

WHAT AGENTS BRING TO THE DISCUSSION

The first step in choosing Medicare coverage is determining the type and cost of healthcare services you need. When we meet with clients, their initial statements often provide clues to their level of healthcare use:

"I haven't seen a doctor in a year and a half."

"I see several specialists."

"I just got over a bout with breast cancer."

"Both knees need replacement in the next year."

"I take several medications and they are expensive."

"I use holistic medicine as much as possible."

We dig deeper by asking questions like:

- Do you travel out of state for extended periods of time?
- Who is your primary care doctor and what specialists do you use?
- Do you have copays with your current plan?
- Are you ok with getting referrals from your primary?
- Do you use a network and how is that working for you?
- Do you have an idea of how much you want to pay for a plan premium?
- What do your friends say about Medicare?
- How important is having a fitness plan with your Medicare?

CMS doesn't want agents prying into clients' lives and digging into their health histories, so that means clients need to volunteer information. Most do because they want a plan that works. All agents are committed—and legally bound—to protect a client's personal and health information.

SCOPE OF APPOINTMENT

Before an agent presents MA, SUPP, and Part D plans, he or she will ask you to sign a Scope of Appointment (SOA). It's a CMS requirement that helps prevent abuse. It doesn't commit you to anything but allows the agent to move forward and talk about the plans. There are electronic methods for signing the form. The SOA has boxes you will check or initial to indicate what you will talk about: MA plans, SUPPs, or Part D plans.

During a plan analysis, we go over:

- Each plan's Summary of Benefits, with explanations of copays and coinsurance
- Part D including tiers, deductibles, copays, coinsurance, and the Donut Hole
- Star ratings
- Differences between MA plans and SUPPs
- Enrollment periods
- How to disenroll or change plans
- HMO and PPO networks
- Added benefits such as vison, hearing, fitness, and dental
- Appeals and grievances

We also relate that agents get paid by insurance companies and do not represent Medicare. We caution that no agent should use superlative terms about a plan or pressure you to enroll. And we point you to language translators if needed.

During a plan assessment, we cover a lot of ground including explaining odd language and unfamiliar terminology. Why? To make sure you, the consumer, get clear and accurate information, develop an adequate understanding of your choices, and are not dealing with a high-pressure salesperson. And we are always available to answer follow-up questions.

A TIP FROM PROFESSOR MEDICARE

Agents or company representatives who work for only one insurance company are known as "captive agents." They can present their companies' plans and no others. What this means is that you will not learn about other plans available in your area. Be very careful in dealing with "captive agents."

As brokers, we present a full menu of plans so you can find the one that fits your needs. Since the commissions are virtually identical for MA plans, there is no reason for us to pressure you to choose one plan over another.

WORK WITH PROFESSOR MEDICARE

We are never too busy for you or your referrals. After working in the senior market for years, we have seen a wide variety of circumstances and situations. That is not to say we have learned everything there is to know about Medicare and senior healthcare, but it takes a lot to surprise us. In 2020, we opened **Professor Medicare's Medicare Resource Center** in Boulder.

We would enjoy working with you and your friends. Here are the states we can serve:

Colorado	New Mexico
Alabama	North Carolina
Alaska	Ohio
Arizona	Oregon
Georgia	Pennsylvania
Kansas	South Dakota
Kentucky	Texas
Michigan	Washington

BUSINESS PROFESSIONALS

Besides providing one-on-one Medicare consultations, we also do presentations and workshops with a variety of professionals and organizations in our community. We work with healthcare organizations, providers, municipalities, educational institutions, CPAs, property and casualty insurance agents, financial planners, and anyone who serves the senior community.

SPEAKING ENGAGEMENTS

If your group or organization would like to schedule an informative Medicare meeting, please give us a thirty-day heads-up.

THE BOOK

If you'd like to purchase *Professor Medicare's Easy Guide to Medicare,* we offer discounts for 20 or more copies.

CALL OR EMAIL US

Donna Ludington: 303-882-1891

donna@professormedicare.com

Craig Stout: 303-885-2725

prof@professormedicare.com

Aidan Stout: 303-999-8523

aidan@professormedicare.com

Or, go to our website *www.professormedicare.com* and request a consultation.

SUMMARY

Although this book can prepare you to make informed choices about Medicare coverage, it can be helpful to go over things with an agent. Experience has taught us what to ask to determine your needs, and our expertise allows us to put together the perfect combination of services. Your information is always kept confidential.

Because they are not affiliated with any particular plan, independent brokers present the full range of options and never pressure you to choose one over another. You can be assured that you are getting an unbiased, impartial review of your needs.

Here is what might be the best reason to consult an agent: working with an expert guide can eliminate your anxiety about making such an important choice.

We hope you'll choose *Professor Medicare*.

CHAPTER QUESTIONS

1. Is there a fee to work with a Medicare agent?
2. True or false: During an appointment, the agent will discuss the differences between Medicare Advantage plans and Supplements.
3. Why should you be wary of meeting with a "captive agent"?
4. Does *Professor Medicare* do presentations to community groups?
5. How can you request a consultation with *Professor Medicare?*

CHAPTER 16

YEARLY UPDATES

We are using 2022 updates for this edition. Medicare may have yearly updates for the following items:

- Part A premium and deductible
- Part B premium and deductible
- Part D deductible
- IRMAA income levels/assessments
- LIS income limits

We will post those changes yearly on our site: *www.ProfessorMedicare.com/book*.

For state income levels for Medicare Savings Plans, we will list Colorado but no other states. Go to your state's SHIP site https://www.medicare.gov/contacts/ to track changes.

A FEW THOUGHTS GOING FORWARD

Congratulations! You finished the book. Our wish is that you have a better understanding of Medicare and how it applies to you.

Just a week ago Craig met with a prospective client who will turn 65 in three months. She was full of questions and opinions. Some of her ideas were based on what friends had told her about Medicare. After sorting through the rubbish, malarkey, and fictions, she calmed down and was able to grasp what was best for her specific situation. Craig advised her that it is wonderful to have friends willing to help, but they should temper their empathy with sound Medicare knowledge and facts. We all have different needs regarding our health and healthcare. What is good for one is not necessarily good for another.

One reason people struggle to understand Medicare is the voluminous stream of information that bombards you when you turn 64 and does not stop. It is truly difficult to separate the signal from the noise. This book will help you do just that. By compressing millions of Medicare-related words into a little over 150 pages, we give you a clear path to making the best healthcare decision for your needs. It's that simple.

Let's look again at the Four Questions-Your **Map to Medicare:**

1. When do I enroll in Medicare?
2. Do I stay with Original Medicare only and add a Part D drug plan? At what cost?
3. Do I enroll in a Medicare Advantage plan that includes/does not include Part D? At what cost?
4. Do I stay with Original Medicare and add a Medigap/Supplement plan and Part D plan? At what cost?

If you get distracted and need to get back on course regarding your Medicare choices, just reread the questions or give us a call.

Here's to your perfect health and longevity!

ABOUT THE AUTHORS

Craig Stout and Donna Ludington are partners in business, life, and joy.

Through their business, *Professor Medicare,* Craig and Donna help seniors digest the alphabet soup that is today's Medicare. The terminology, number of options, and tiny details can overwhelm anyone who tries to go it alone. But as independent insurance brokers, Craig and Donna turn that multitude of choices to their clients' advantage. They shop multiple carriers and plans to find the best combination of healthcare and drug coverage for each individual. Their combined 20 years of experience helps them advise those who want to keep working after 65, determine the best high-use prescription plans, and recommend out-of-area coverage. Plus, *Professor Medicare* educates clients about Medicare's numerous enrollment periods in case situations change.

Active in their Metro Denver, Colorado, business community, Craig and Donna share their expertise as featured speakers at senior centers, community and business meetings, and national conferences.

Before launching *Professor Medicare,* the couple owned Sumitra Gift and Jewelry, a wholesale distributorship. It began with a desire to create something together as newlyweds. They purchased a small cache of Peruvian jewelry from a relative and started selling to small retailers. The business grew to gift/jewelry and clothing showrooms, two warehouses, and multiple employees and road reps. They had a national following in the New Age market.

With their son's birth in 1996, Craig and Donna embarked on a new path. They sold their Sumitra businesses and moved to San Diego County, California, where Craig ran a small professional theatre and Donna managed residential properties. Later Craig worked at the largest realtor training company in the United States.

In 2010, the couple returned to their beloved Denver and their healthcare roots. They had met while working at the Pritikin Longevity Center in Los Angeles. Donna's physician parents managed a hospital in Bangkok, where she was born. She accompanied her father into the northern Thailand hill country to treat people who rarely saw a doctor. At eleven Donna served as her father's surgical assistant.

Veering away from healthcare, Donna established an English language school in southern Thailand. In Los Angeles, she worked as a therapist for abandoned and abused children for over ten years. She also served as the center's director. Craig, too, pursued non-healthcare ventures. After college and a stint in the U.S. Navy, the native Kentuckian worked as a professional actor.

Now, Craig and Donna have come full circle, all their life experiences folding into a career they see as a calling—helping people safeguard their physical and economic health by making the right healthcare choices. That business is about to get a shot in the arm from their greatest joy—their son, Aidan. A recent graduate of Ohio Wesleyan University, Aidan honored in business and played soccer at the winningest program in collegiate history. He will bring great energy and resourcefulness to the independent brokerage, ensuring that *Professor Medicare* will continue to help seniors for years to come.

APPENDIX

A. Chapter Questions and Answers
B. Organizations Linked to Medicare
C. Medicare Publications
D. Special Enrollment Periods (SEP)
E. Fines: Part B, Part D, Appealing a Fine

A. Chapter Questions and Answers

Chapter 1

1. When was Medicare signed into law? **1965**
2. Does Part A cover outpatient surgery? **No, B does**
3. What Part covers X-rays? **B**
4. What organization oversees Medicare? **The Centers for Medicare Services (CMS)**
5. How can you help protect Medicare from cuts? **Contact your Members of Congress**

Chapter 2

1. What is the difference between a *part* and a *plan?* **Parts are the 4 Medicare parts—A, B, D, and D; plans are insurer-created coverage to bundle with or supplement Original Medicare**
2. What does Part B cover? **Physician and outpatient services**
3. How many Supplements will be offered in 2022? **9**

4. What is a copay? **A fixed amount you pay at the time of service**

5. What happens after you meet your Maximum Out-of-Pocket? **Your health plan pays 100% for the rest of the year**

Chapter 3

1. When was prescription drug coverage added to Medicare? **2006**

2. Once you have paid into Medicare for 10 years or 40 quarters, what is your Part A premium? **$0**

3. What is the Part B deductible? **$233**

4. What covers you if you are admitted to a hospital? **Part A**

5. Does Part B cover hearing aids? **No**

Chapter 4

1. When is Annual Enrollment (AEP)? **October 15–December 7**

2. Do you need a referral if you have a PPO? **No**

3. When do companies communicate their Annual Notice of Changes? **September**

4. When is OEP and what can you do at that time? **Open Enrollment Period is January 1–March 31. You can move from one MA plan to another or move back to Original Medicare**

5. Do you need a primary care physician with an HMO? **Yes**

Chapter 5

1. Will Plan F be sold in 2022? **Only if you turned 65 before January 1, 2020.**

2. What is Issue-Aged pricing? **Your SUPP premium is based on your age when your policy is issued; it may go up in a "statewide increase"**

3. Will your Supplement premium stay the same? **No. These change yearly**

4. Can a company raise your premium if you have too many claims? **No**

5. Do Supplements include drug coverage? **No**

Chapter 6

1. Do I need to answer health questions to change my Medicare Advantage plan? **No**

2. Do Supplements have a lot of extra benefits like Medicare Advantage plans? **No, although a few have Silver Sneakers/Silver and Fit**

3. Do most Medicare Advantage plans have a Part B deductible? **Rarely**

4. Can I get a Medicare Advantage plan without a network? **No**

5. If I just had a heart attack and want to change my Supplement, would that be easy to do? **No, you would most likely be denied coverage**

Chapter 7

1. When will you find out about yearly changes for your Part D plan? **September via the Annual Notice of Changes**
2. Do all plans charge a deductible? **No**
3. What costs more: A Tier 2 or Tier 4 medication? **Tier 4**
4. Will there be a copay for a shingles vaccination? **Yes**
5. Do all Medicare Advantage plans have a Part D? **No. MAPD includes drugs but MA, most PFFS, and MSA plans do not have Part D**

Chapter 8

1. How long is the Initial Enrollment Period? **7 Months**
2. Where do you enroll in Medicare when turning 65? **Online at *www.ssa.gov* or *www.Medicare.gov*, by calling Social Security, or visiting a Social Security office**
3. What is the Part B monthly premium? **$170.10 a month (but more for higher incomes)**
4. Can you change plans during the year? **Yes** When? **During AEP or OEP**
5. What is 5-Star Enrollment? **You can drop your MA or SUPP and enroll in a 5-star MA anytime during the year, but only once a year**

Chapter 9

1. If you already receive Social Security, do you have to sign up for Medicare? **No, you will be enrolled automatically**

2. If you plan to keep working after 65, can you keep your employer health plan? **If your company has fewer than 20 full-time employees, you must enroll in Medicare A and B; if more than 20, you may keep your employer plan until you retire**

3. When you leave an employer health plan and begin Medicare, what two forms do you need to file? **CMS Forms L564 and 40B.**

4. What is the timeline for enrolling in Medicare when leaving an employer plan? **8 months to enroll in Medicare Parts A and B; 2 months for C and D**

5. How do you prove your employer drug coverage was "creditable"? **Ask your employer's benefits administrator to provide, on company letterhead, your dates of coverage from age 65**

Chapter 10

1. Can you change your Supplement Plan G to a Plan N whenever you want? **Yes**

2. Can you change your Part D when you switch Supplements? **Only during AEP from Oct 15– Dec 7**

3. If you just qualified for a Low-Income Subsidy, can you change MA plans? **Yes**

4. My neighbor told me I can change my drug plan during the Open Enrollment Period from January 1–March 31. Is this true? **No, only during AEP**

5. Can I change from a Supplement to a Medicare Advantage plan during the Annual Enrollment Period in the fall? **Yes**

Chapter 11

1. True or False: 75% of retirees have a retirement strategy. **False. Only 46% have a strategy.**

2. Can anyone qualify for a Low-Income Subsidy? **No, you must be below certain income and resource levels.**

3. Will the QMB level of a Medicare Savings Program pay for the Part B premium? **Yes, and more.**

4. Does an auto or home count as a resource when applying for extra help? **No, not if you live in your home.**

5. Where should one apply for a Medicare Savings Program? **At your County Department of Human Services.**

Chapter 12

1. If I am applying for Medicare in 2022, will they look at my 2019 tax return? **No, your 2020 return**

2. My household income is $150,000. Will I have an IRMAA charge? **No, you are under $182,000**

3. Is my income my AGI? **No, it's your MAGI**

4. How much would my IRMAA be for Part B and Part D if our joint income is $300,000? **Part B is $442.30 and Part D is $51.70 for a total of $494.**

5. Can I appeal an IRMAA charge online? **Yes, or in writing or at a Social Security office**

Chapter 13

1. Where can you access your claims history online? ***www.mymedicare.gov***
2. Is PACE for anyone on Medicare? **No, only for those who are frail and eligible for a nursing home**
3. Is there a charge for flu shots? **No**
4. If you have a back operation and can't move enough to go to therapy sessions, what Medicare program can you use? **Home Health Care**
5. What part of Medicare covers you during an "observation" hospital stay? **Part B**

Chapter 14

1. If I think I was overcharged $100 for an office visit, should I file an appeal or a grievance? **Appeal**
2. The receptionist at my dermatologist said she was tired of dealing with old people and their brown spots. Can I file a grievance? **Yes**
3. If I am in hospital and was turned down for an operation, can my doctor get a fast appeal? **Yes, your doctor can request an *expedited appeal***
4. If there was a coding error on my bill, should I immediately file an appeal? **No, first call the office**
5. The company that delivers my oxygen is never on time and I often must call several times to get it. Is this grounds for an appeal or a grievance? **Grievance**

Chapter 15

1. Is there a fee to work with a Medicare agent? **No**
2. True or false: During an appointment, the agent will discuss the differences between Medicare Advantage plans and Supplements. **True**
3. Why should you be wary of meeting with a "captive agent"? **A captive agent can only present his or her company's plans, not the full range of plans**
4. Does *Professor Medicare* do presentations to community groups? **Yes**
5. How can you request a consultation with *Professor Medicare?* **Request a consultation at** ***www.professormedicare.com***

B. Organizations

Medicare

www.medicare.gov

800-633-4227

CMS

www.cms.gov

Social Security

www.ssa.gov

800-772-1213

SHIP—Colorado

888-696-7213

Professor Medicare

www.professormedicare.com

858-689-7445/303-885-2725/303-882-1891/303-999-8523

C. Publications

You can find these publications at *www.medicare.gov:*

- Choosing a Medigap Policy: A Guide to Health Insurance for People with Medicare
- Learning What Medicare Covers and How Much You Pay
- Medicare & You 2022
- Medicare Appeals
- Medicare Premiums: Rules for Higher-Income Beneficiaries
- Medicare Rights & Protections
- Protecting Yourself & Medicare from Fraud
- Quick Facts About Programs of All-Inclusive Care for the Elderly
- Understanding Medicare Advantage Plans

D. Special Enrollment Periods (SEP)

Special Enrollment Periods let you make changes to Medicare Advantage and Part D plans. If you move, lose other coverage, or experience other major changes in your life, you may qualify for an SEP. Since the list is extensive, the best way to check on your qualification for an SEP is to go to the page linked to Medicare.gov: *https://www.medicare.gov/sign-up-change-plans/when-can-i-join-a-health-or-drug-plan/special-circumstances-special-enrollment-periods.*

E. Fines

Part B Fine

Medicare assesses a fine for a lapse in Part B coverage. The fine is 10% of the Part B premium for every full year you didn't have Part B. If the premium is $170.10, then 10% of that is $17.01. You add that to the base premium every month, multiplied by the number of years without Part B.

For example, imagine you are 67 and did not enroll in Medicare Part B when you were first eligible. You have gone two years without Part B coverage.

Monthly Part B premium	$170.10
Fine: 10% of $170.10 = $17.01 x 2 years without Part B	+ 34.02
New premium forever	$204.12

Your fine is 10% of the $170.10 Part B premium, which equals $17.01. Multiplied by 2 years, the monthly fine equals $34.02. That $34.02 gets added to your Part B premium, for a total of $204.12 every month forever after. The only way to avoid the fine is to become eligible for Medicaid or another low-income assistance program.

Part D Fine

If you don't enroll in a Part D plan during IEP, you may be subject to a Part D fine. You could owe a late enrollment penalty if, for any continuous period of 63 days or more after your IEP ends, you go without one of these:

- A Medicare Prescription Drug Plan (Part D)
- A Medicare Advantage Plan (Part C) (like an HMO or PPO) with Part D
- Another Medicare health plan that offers Medicare prescription drug coverage
- Creditable prescription drug coverage

Medicare determines the penalty by multiplying 1% of the "national base beneficiary premium" ($33.37 for 2022) times the number of full, uncovered months you didn't have Part D or creditable coverage. The monthly premium is rounded to the nearest $.10 and added to your monthly Part D premium. For example, if you have not had Part D for 12 months and enroll in a plan to start in 2022 your monthly fine is $.33 x 12 months, equaling $3.96.

Remember, Medicare adds this fine to your Part D plan premium every month. Also, the national base beneficiary premium could increase or increase each year, so your penalty amount may change yearly.

What if you have a Medicare Advantage plan with a $0 premium? In that case, they will only bill you for the Part D fine.

Appealing a Fine

If you object to any fine or ruling regarding your Medicare coverage, you can appeal it. CMS has contracted with MAXIMUS as the agency to handle and rule on all appeals for Parts A, C, and D.

If you want to appeal a Part B ruling, contact Social Security or Medicare.

If you receive a letter from your Part D plan requesting proof of coverage, there will be additional information regarding the appeals process. Be sure to read everything and meet the deadlines.

GLOSSARY

Medicare Terms and Abbreviations

A	Abbreviation for Medicare Part A/ hospitalization
ACA	Affordable Care Act—healthcare reform enacted in 2010
AEP	Annual Enrollment Period October 15– December 7
ANOC	Annual Notice of Changes
B	Abbreviation for Medicare Part B/health care
C	Abbreviation for Medicare Part C/Medicare Advantage
CMS	Centers for Medicare and Medicaid Services— Medicare's ruling body
COBRA	Insurance that extends your coverage after you leave employment
Cost Plan	A Medicare Advantage plan
D	Abbreviation for Medicare Part D/drug plans
Coinsurance	The % you pay for a covered service
Copay	A fixed amount you pay at the time of service
Creditable Drug Coverage	Group, individual, student, children's, or government healthcare plans
Deductible	A fixed amount you pay out of pocket before your plan starts paying

Donut Hole	A gap in coverage when you pay more
EOC	Evidence of Coverage notice
ESRD	End-stage renal disease
Formulary	A tiered list of generic and brand name drugs your insurer uses to set prices
GEP	General Enrollment Period January 1–March 31
GI	Guaranteed Issue right—situations that guarantee you coverage
HMO	Health Maintenance Organization
ICEP	Initial Coverage Enrollment Period
IEP	Initial Enrollment Period—7-month period: 3 months before birth month + birth month + 3 months following
IRMAA	Income-Related Monthly Adjustment Amount
LIS	Low-Income Subsidy for Part D assistance
MA	Medicare Advantage plan without Part D coverage
MAPD	Medicare Advantage plan with Part D coverage
MAX OOP	MAX OOP—The cap on the amount you must pay for services in a year
Medigap	Medicare Supplement plan
MSA	Medicare Savings Account—a Medicare Advantage plan
MSN	Medicare Summary Notice
MSP	Medicare Savings Programs—state-run programs that assist qualifying individuals with premiums, copays, and coinsurance

OEP	Open Enrollment Period January 1–March 31
Original Medicare	Medicare Parts A and B
PACE	Program of All-Inclusive Care for the Elderly
PDP	Prescription Drug Plan
PFFS	Private Fee-for-Service—a Medicare Advantage plan
POS	Point-of-Service plan
PPO	Preferred Provider Organization
RPPO	Regional Preferred Provider Organization
Premium	The amount you pay (usually monthly) for health insurance
SNP	Special Needs Plan—CSNP = Chronic Care / DSNP = Dual Eligible (Medicare and Medicaid) / ISNP = Institutionalized Plan
SOA	Scope of Appointment—a form that gives your agent permission to discuss plans with you
SUPP	Medicare Supplement plan
Supplement	Medicare Supplement plan
TROOP	True Out-of-Pocket Costs

BIBLIOGRAPHY

"An Overview of Medicare." *Medicare.* Kaiser Family Foundation. February 13, 2019. https://www.kff.org/medicare/issue-brief/an-overview-of-medicare/.

"Anticipated Congressional Proposals to Cut Medicare, Medicaid and Social Security." National Committee to Preserve Social Security & Medicare. January 16, 2018. https://www.ncpssm.org/documents/general-archives-2018/anticipated-congressional-proposals-cut-medicare-medicaid-social-security-2018/.

Gleitzman, Morris. *Then* (New York: Square Fish, 2013).

Haeder, Simon F. "Why the US Has Higher Drug Prices than Other Countries." *The Conversation.* February 7, 2019. https://theconversation.com/why-the-us-has-higher-drug-prices-than-other-countries-111256.

Johnson, Lyndon B. "Remarks with President Truman at the Signing in Independence of the Medicare Bill." *Social Security: History.* July 30, 1965. https://www.ssa.gov/history/lbjstmts.html.

Luhby, Tami. "How Trump Wants to Whack Medicare and Medicaid Spending." *CNN Politics.* March 3, 2019. https://www.cnn.com/2019/03/13/politics/medicare-medicaid-trump-budget/index.html.

Mole, Beth. "Years after Mylan's Epic EpiPen Price Hikes, it Finally Gets a Generic Rival." *Ars Technica*. August 17, 2018. https://arstechnica.com/science/2018/08/fda-approves-generic-version-of-mylans-600-epipens-but-the-price-is-tbd/.

Nall, Rachel. "How Much Does Hepatitis C Treatment Cost?" *Medical News Today*. November 21, 2018. https://www.medicalnewstoday.com/articles/323767.php.

Oberlander, Jonathan. "The Political History of Medicare." *Generations*. American Society on Aging. Summer, 2015. https://www.asaging.org/blog/political-history-medicare.

"Opioid Addiction." *Genetics Home Reference*. NIH U.S. National Library of Medicine. October 29, 2019. https://ghr.nlm.nih.gov/condition/opioid-addiction#statistics.

Rappold, R. Scott. "Families Cross Borders in Search for Affordable Insulin." *WebMD*. July 18, 2019. https://www.webmd.com/diabetes/news/20190718/spiking-insulin-costs-put-patients-in-brutal-bind.

Roberts, Danielle K. "The Deadly Costs of Insulin." *AJMC*. June 10, 2019. https://www.ajmc.com/contributor/danielle-roberts/2019/06/the-deadly-costs-of-insulin.

Silverman, Ed. "Insulin Prices Could Be Much Lower and Drug Makers Would Still Make Healthy Profits." *Business Insider*. September 26, 2018.

https://www.businessinsider.com/insulin-prices-could-be-much-lower-and-drug-makers-would-still-make-healthy-profits-2018-9.

Zelizer, Julian E. "How Medicare Was Made." *The New Yorker*. February 15, 2015. https://www.newyorker.com/news-desk/medicare-made.

Made in the USA
Middletown, DE
19 February 2022

61471586R00111